Contents

The Creation of the National Health Service

A study of pressure groups and a major social policy decision

by Arthur J. Willcocks
Senior Lecturer in Social Science
University of Nottingham

LONDON
ROUTLEDGE AND KEGAN PAUL
NEW YORK: THE HUMANITIES PRESS

First published 1967
by Routledge and Kegan Paul Limited
Broadway House, 68-74 Carter Lane
London, E.C.4

Printed in Great Britain
by Northumberland Press Limited
Gateshead on Tyne

The Creation of the National Health Service

LIBRARY OF SOCIAL POLICY
AND ADMINISTRATION

GENERAL EDITOR: DR. KATHLEEN JONES
Professor of Social Administration
University of York

Books in the Series include

Mental Health Services—split between domiciliary and institutional care—little special consideration of this service.

The erosion of early plans—the failure to achieve administrative unification—the gradual splintering of administration. The filling in of detail from one plan to the next.

The balance sheet of successes and failures for the groups—the great success of the professional skilled groups.

The pressures today—the changing outline of these pressures—new groups and pressures—growing specialization and the role of the layman—the professional man in a nationalized service.

A note on the sources used—recommendations for further reading.

General editor's introduction

The Library of Social Policy and Administration is designed to provide short texts suitable for the needs of Social Studies students in universities and other centres of higher education. They will also be of use to administrators in the social services, practising social workers, and others whose work brings them into contact with the developing field of social service.

The Library will provide studies in depth rather than surveys of the whole field of social policy, and each volume will be complete in itself. Some will be studies of the British Social Services. Others will offer accounts of social policy in other countries, and provide material for comparative study. A third group will consist of case-studies in the processes of social policy.

Dr. Willcocks's analysis of the Creation of the National Health Service is such a case-study. He is concerned with one piece of social legislation—the National Health Service Act of 1946—and with the political, economic and social forces which shaped it. War-time needs had forced the fragmented Health Services of the 1930s into temporary fusion. There was general agreement that a national system should be set up, and the publication of the Beveridge

Report in 1942, which assumed the existence of a National Health Service as fundamental to the creation of a system of social security, marked the beginning of an intense public interest in this important area of social policy. Should general practitioners be salaried, or preserve the independence of professional standards and status? Should the great voluntary hospitals stand outside the scheme, or come into it—and if so, on what basis? Could continuity of care be maintained in a tripartite system? What would the role of the local authorities be if a separate Hospitals Service were created?

Questions such as these were hotly debated for four years. The policies of the major political parties, the interests of medical and other professional groups, the traditions evolved over many years of trial and error by local authorities and central government departments all played a part in the shaping of a major piece of legislation. So did the views of the man in the street—now not only the potential patient, but also, as a tax-paying citizen, the financial backer of the new service. The interaction of individuals and groups in creating a viable policy out of conflicting interests, and in solving difficult technical problems of administration, many of them without precedent, makes a fascinating story. It is valuable not only in providing a background of understanding to present conflicts and tensions within the Health Service, but as a study of the processes of social action at work in a democratic society.

KATHLEEN JONES

NOTE

Throughout this book detailed references to Hansard, to the many journals and group documents used are not given. Instead, major references and useful sources for further reading are given in the Bibliography. The full documentation of this study can be found in the author's Ph.D. thesis 'Interest Groups and the National Health Service Act, 1946', lodged with the Librarian, University of Birmingham.

Preface

Most of the debts of thanks that I owe relate to the original Ph.D. thesis which was written in the mid-1950s and on which this book is based. Many health service and pressure group officials at that time gave me much help in the loan of publications and material and in giving up time for discussion with me. My prime thanks for that thesis were due to my supervisor, Mr. Henry Maddick, now Senior Lecturer in the University of Birmingham. No research student can accurately measure his debt to his supervisor: mine, I know, was a large one.

This book, coming many years after the original thesis, owes much to the many officials of the service who during these years have always welcomed me and allowed me to take part in their conferences.

To my wife who has had to live with my interest in the National Health Service all her married life, I owe more than can be expressed.

If despite all the help and encouragement, weaknesses, errors and omissions remain, I alone am to blame.

A.J.W.

1
Introduction

'Case studies never "prove" anything' wrote one recent author on health services in this country (Eckstein 1960), adding that 'their purpose is to illustrate generalizations which are established otherwise, or to direct attention towards such generalizations'. This book is such a case study and has two aims—to direct attention towards generalizations that might be made about social policy decisions and the way they are taken, and to add a measure of understanding for the student of today's National Health Service by looking in some detail at an aspect of its creation. To meet these aims, the detail must be supplemented both by some comments on the sorts of generalization towards which studies of social policy decisions might be directing attention, and by a sketch outline of the historical development of health services within which the episode considered here must be set.

Social policy decisions

That there is ample scope for lengthy semantic discussion on what is implied by the phrase 'social policy decisions' and on each of its three words, the reader would do well to remember. For this study, however, we take policy decisions to mean the decisions of government on matters of some consequence (e.g. the creation of a health service or the remodelling of the social security system) taken with the express or implied purpose of obliterating, reducing or ameliorating social problems. In saying this we perhaps merely transfer the semantic argument to 'social problems', but short-circuiting any such argument, we define a social problem as a set of phenomena of a social kind which is recognized by government as creating a problem and about which it seeks to do something.

If, therefore, we assume that social policy decisions are governmental decisions of consequence about recognized social problems, then the study of social policy decisions involves at least four (and probably more) questions of some importance. What is it that creates a social problem is a question clearly of fundamental importance as the mainspring of the need for social policies. Perhaps of less importance, but still of interest to the student, is the question of what makes a social problem come to be recognized as such by a government. Closely related to this latter question is one which asks what are the influences and factors that make a government do something about one particular social problem and not another, and make them do something at one point in time and not another. This leads finally to the question about the content of the decision as expressed in Acts of Parliament, new administrative structures and the like: what are the factors that influence the content of the decision? In this study, this last question in relation to the National Health Service Act, 1946 is the one to which our main effort is directed, but partial answers to the others will appear from time to time.

Factors influencing decisions and decision making

The factors which are likely to influence the sort of decisions taken can be listed and the reader may wish to decide for himself whether the concentration here on the pressure group as an influencing factor does a disservice to the other factors. In a country which prides itself on its democracy a factor of importance ought surely to be public opinion. What public opinion is, or rather what public opinions, in the plural, are is not always easy to discover for there is no formalized system for their expression except through the democratic process of election. Of more importance, therefore, in influencing social policy will be the elected members of Parliament and the political parties they group themselves in : that a change of political party in control will change the general tenor of policy decisions, even if only marginally, is clearly a fact of political life. The political colour of government is then one important factor influencing decisions.

Within Parliament and the parties, the influence of individual members of groups of members can sometimes be traced, but the members themselves seem rarely to respond to sectional or specialized interests in any major way unless the issues are taken by the political party of which they are members. The very generalized nature of election on a geographical constituency basis, and the generalized operation of the political party makes it extremely difficult for specialized groups—e.g. doctors—to press their particular views through Parliament. Instead as society has become more and more specialized and social policy more and more complicated and pervasive of many facets of the national life, groups with special interests or viewpoints have banded together to press their views on the Government, the ministers and their departments, Parliament and wherever else seems important. The decisions to be taken on the shape of the proposed National Health Service were of such a complicated nature and the number of specialized groups involved so very many, that this case-study of the designing the shape of the service and of the part the groups played in this process seeks to throw some light on pressure groups and social policy decisions.

Although, of all the factors which may influence social policy decisions, pressure groups are singled out here, this is not to discount many others that may, and, in this case often did, operate. These other factors may include the views of the civil service administrators, the findings of Royal Commissions and Committees of Enquiry, research studies and the campaigns of individual or groups of reformers. They may also include many other less easily identifiable factors which may often repay serious investigation. The factors thus are many, and pressure groups are only part of the total picture; our claim here is not that these groups are of paramount importance in all decisions, or, indeed, in the case of this Act, but rather that any account of the writing of the National Health Service Act without reference to the role of these groups is, at least, incomplete if not inaccurate. We are not trying to show the role of the pressure groups in identifying the problem (the need for improved health service provision) although many groups undoubtedly played a part in this process: rather the aim is to show how, once the decision to create a National Health Service was taken, pressure groups played an important part in the decision-making process on the shape of the service.

In doing this we are staking a claim for the importance of what may be termed political realities rather than abstract principles in social policy decisions. 'Many of those who have drawn up paper plans for the health services', said Aneurin Bevan in introducing his Bill to Parliament in 1946, 'appear to have followed the dictates of abstract principles and not the concrete requirements of the actual situation as it exists'. Pressure groups are part of the 'actual situation' as is public opinion and the views of the party in the majority position in the Commons, so we shall conclude, with *The Lancet*, that the Act derived 'much more from the long discussion between the profession and the Minister of Health than it (did) from any doctrinaire idea of . . . Minister's political party'.

Having made the major decision to create a health service, the Minister concerned was faced with a range of alternative means to use to design it. He might, for example, have wished to retain the existing administrative structures, to modify them and their powers or to start afresh. The decision he took and wrote into his plan might have coincided with the views of one pressure group whilst being opposed to that of another. He might have decided along the lines he did because of what he and his advisers considered to be the relative strengths of the pressure groups and what they could offer or withhold, or he may have been convinced of the logic of one side's argument and failed to see it in the other's viewpoint. His decisions therefore might have been a concession to pressure or a rational convincement to a point of view, or there may have been elements of both in his decision. Without access to his papers and his advisers, one can rarely be sure which was the true answer. In making this study, no access to such papers or persons was granted, so here, without assuming either solution, we simply point out the views of the groups and their successes measured in terms of how much of their views found their way into the National Health Service Act, 1946. Rationality or the big stick, logic or concession are not of importance here: the resultant shape of the service is what is sought.

Thus far, we have outlined something of a speculative

framework of thought and defined the aims—a case-study of the successes of pressure groups is one legislative expression of a social policy decision. The discussion is limited to the Act of 1946 and not to the regulations that flowed from it (although these would repay further study along these lines); the Act of 1946 itself is limited to England and Wales, the Scottish counterpart following a year later with some modifications. We can now in the next chapter sketch in some of the specific detail of this case study.

2

The Act and the pressure groups

This chapter provides firstly a summary of the main provisions of the National Health Service Act 1946 together with a chronology of the main events leading up to it. These events are presented in tabular form below. Finally the chapter ends with a look at the pressure groups concerned and their views.

CHRONOLOGY OF MAJOR EVENTS LEADING TO
NATIONAL HEALTH SERVICE ACT 1946

1939	Creation of Emergency Medical Services as part of war-time measures.
9th October 1941	Announcement by Ernest Brown, Minister of Health of
	1. Decision to create a national hospital service after the war.
	2. Survey of existing hospital facilities.

November 1942   Publication of Beveridge Report 'Social Insurance and Allied Services' and its recommendation of a comprehensive health service.

February 1943   Government acceptance of planning a health service. Negotiations begin.

March 1943   The Minister reveals his plans (The Brown Plan).

December 1943   Willink replaces Brown as Minister of Health.

February 1944   White Paper 'A National Health Service' published (The White Paper).

Summer 1944   D-day landings in Normandy—negotiations suspended.

March/April 1945   Willink devises a revised plan (The Willink Plan).

July 1945   General Election—Labour Victory. Bevan becomes Minister.

March 1946   National Health Service Bill—read a First time and published. (N.H.S. Bill)

November 1946   National Health Service Bill receives Royal Assent and becomes an Act.

(The phrases in brackets are the short titles by which the various plans are referred to in the text.)

(A) The National Health Service Act

The National Health Service, as created by the Act of 1946,

is a comprehensive service covering almost all forms of medical care which are freely (or almost freely) available to all irrespective of class, sex, colour, domicile, race or membership of insurance schemes. In the main independently financed, it has no connection with the social security system (unlike the health schemes in many other countries) and its services are not limited to those who contribute to that security system. (There are separate health service contributions payable with the national insurance weekly contribution but these give no special entitlement to or relationship between the services). Its finances come, except for this special levy, from the general exchequer—i.e. national taxes, and from local rates. Where the patient pays at all, the charges apply only to less costly services, e.g. dentistry, and home-helps. It is, therefore, a community financed service available to all without means test and only rarely after a charge: it is available to all but not compulsorily so. Doctors both in hospitals and in the general practitioner services are given the right to spend part of their time in private practice (even using private beds in the state hospitals) and the patient has the right to choose this private treatment if he so desires, and, of course, can afford to do so.

The central administrative responsibility 'to promote the establishment of a comprehensive health service' belongs to the Minister of Health (Lindsey 1962). He is advised in this duty by a Central Health Services Council, representative of the main groups in the service and by specialized Standing Advisory Committees. The membership of the council, which is set out in the First Schedule of the Act, consists of 41 members. Of these 15 are doctors together with another 6 ex-officio medical representatives, 5 have hospital management experience, 5 have local government experience, 3 are dentists, 2 have experience in mental health services, 2 are nurses, 1 a midwife and 2 are pharmacists. As we shall see the exact composition of this Council came to be of some importance in the discussions on the proposed service.

The Ministry of Health, despite the title, was also concerned, in 1948, with housing and supervisory local government duties. In 1951, after Aneurin Bevan's resignation, the Ministry was reorganized losing its local government and housing responsibilities, thus becoming something more like its title. In so doing, it undoubtedly lost esteem and, with it, Cabinet status.

Away from the national centre the Service is, in reality, three separate service organizations only very loosely linked: a tripartite structure which has evoked much discussion since 1948 and is, as we shall see, a monument to the pressure groups' conflicting views. The three sections, which we shall examine briefly in turn, are hospital and specialist services, general practitioner services and local health authority services.

1 Hospital and specialist services

The most spectacular and controversial innovation of the Act was to vest all (or almost all) hospitals, whatever their previous ownership, in the Minister (Section 6). This transfer of ownership made it necessary and possible to design a special administrative structure for the hospital service. Excluding medical teaching hospitals (i.e. those hospitals where medical students are trained) all hospitals were grouped together for administration purposes under a two-tiered structure. The country (England & Wales) is sub-divided into regions (at first 14 but now 15) and in each region a Regional Hospital Board was created. (Section 11.) Approved by the Minister, the Board is responsible for the guidance, planning and control of hospital services in this area. The regions were so drawn as to include at least one medical teaching hospital in each region, a requirement which has produced some odd boundary solutions (e.g. in London). The members of the Board are appointed and not elected, are unpaid and although they include qualified medical men, are not appointed to serve any representative or delegate function.

Each region has subdivided its area and hospitals into smaller groups for day to day administrative control. For each such group, Hospital Management Committees are appointed by the Boards (Section 11), the conditions of membership being similar to those of Board members. The medical teaching hospitals are administratively separate from this system being controlled by Boards of governors. The money to pay for these services comes almost entirely from Exchequer funds (i.e. national taxation), a fact which considerably reduced the power of boards and committees in their dealings with the Ministry. There are however two other sources of finance : one is the distribution among all hospitals of the income from the Hospital Endowments Fund. The Act transferred all hospital endowments (except those of the teaching hospital) to this fund, to even out the uneven distribution of endowment monies, and allowed hospitals to use their income from the fund in a wider way and without the financial controls associated with Exchequer monies. Hence the name 'free monies' often given to this income. The other source of finance, a very small one, is the income from charges levied on those patients who wish to use the private (pay) beds or the partially private (amenity) beds which hospitals may provide (sections 4 and 5).

2 *General practitioner services*

The services covered by this part of the service are the general practitioner, medical and dental services, the

17

general practitioner obstetric services, the pharmaceutical services and, in a somewhat anomalous position, the ophthalmic services. Except in the case of the last mentioned services which are controlled by a temporary structure the Supplementary Ophthalmic Services Committees, these services are the responsibility of Local Executive Councils (Section 31). Unlike the hospital authorities whose administrative boundaries do not necessarily coincide with local government boundaries, executive councils are conterminous in areas with county and county borough councils. These councils are made up of members, some appointed by the professions working in the service in the area, some by the local health authority and a crucial few by the Minister himself. In each case they are unpaid and are similarly placed to hospital members.

Their duties are limited to making arrangements with the doctors, dentists, and the others for the provision of services in their area, to publishing lists of such medical men who are willing to provide services and to being paymaster to these professionals. They are responsible through special committees and subject to ministerial approval for the hearing of and decisions on complaints against the professionals providing services. They have the duty in conjunction with the Medical Practices Committee (Section 34) of appointing new general medical practitioners to their areas and thereby assuring a better geographical distribution of doctors.

Each of the professionals who operate in these services, work as 'independent contractors' in return for either a *per-capita* fee or a fee for services performed. Doctors are paid a yearly sum for each person on their list—i.e. those for whom the doctor has accepted responsibility—irrespective of what they do for them. He (and the patient) have the right to choose or reject one another subject to certain limitations. The dentist, pharmacist and optician, however,

18

does not have to accept such a responsibility—he must agree to be available for National Health Service patients although he is not bound in the same pervasive way as the doctor is. In return, he gets, unlike the doctor, a fee for each service performed, the patient having to make some contribution to the cost. Except for this element, the bulk of the cost of all executive council services comes from the exchequer.

The doctor, but none of the others, has lost the right to buy and sell the goodwill of his practice and the right to work whenever he pleases. The doctor is, thus, more closely linked with the system than the other professions who are not subject to the control of lists, of non-sale of practices, and of limitations on where they may practise.

3 Local authority services

The third part of the service rests with the traditional system of local democracy—the county and county borough councils and is operated in the normal local government way. Local authorities provide, under the Act, maternity and child welfare services, domiciliary midwifery services, district nurses, home helps, ambulances, mental health services outside the hospital system, health centres, and for the after care of illness (a wide permissive clause which can cover many things). These services operate as only one part of the vast range of services provided by major local authorities. The local authorities draw their finances from rates, central government grants, and charges levied in some services on the user.

This, in brief, is the National Health Service—split rather than unified, free but with private practice and including both elective and appointed systems: all in all as odd administrative structure, especially when viewed against early attempts at a simplified but comprehensive administration.

The health services in 1939

The origins of the National Health Service go back over many centuries and present a fascinating history of painful development which for reasons of space cannot be traced here. Much of this history is well documented (e.g. Abel-Smith 1964, Ross 1952, Harris 1946) so that all we need do is to glance briefly at the situation in 1939 and at some of its alleged deficiencies. This is important if the view of one writer is accepted (Eckstein 1959) that the Act of 1946 represents an attempt at rationalization and redistribution rather than a great advance. Whatever may have been the views in 1946, there seems little doubt that its subsequent development lends considerable support to this thesis.

In 1939 hospitals were provided by either local authorities or by voluntary bodies, the local authority hospitals providing some 143,000 beds whilst the more numerous voluntary hospitals, provided fewer beds (about 72,000). The local authorities concentrated in the main on fever, isolation and mental hospitals although after legislation in 1930 they were expanding their work with general hospitals. With statutory responsibilities the local authorities had little option in their choice of patients whilst the voluntary hospitals whose patients either paid (in person or through some insurance system) or were given free treatment, could pick and choose their patients (Abel-Smith 1964). The many hospital authorities rarely co-operated to achieve a rational provision of services in any area.

Under the National Health Insurance Act 1911 (Levy 1944) certain groups of the working population, mainly manual and lower paid workers, could obtain free general practitioner medical services by virtue of their contributions to the scheme. The 'panel' system, as it was known, was operated by local insurance committees who also provided pharmaceutical services for the contributors. In the complicated system of approved societies, some contributors also qualified for the 'additional' benefits of free or reduced cost dentistry and ophthalmic services.

The local authorities were providing, in addition to their hospitals, maternity and child welfare services and some of the other services which remain their responsibility today (Wilson 1946). These duties were not, however, limited only to county and county borough councils as is the case under the 1946 Act, but were the responsibility, often, of the smaller local authorities.

The deficiencies of 1939

The total picture of these services in the pre-war days was described by commentators of the period as one of a 'bewildering variety of agencies' (P.E.P. 1937) and 'complicated and somewhat inchoate' (Newsholme 1932). The administration of the services was carried on by many organizations but was the overall responsibility of no one body. The Ministry of Health, a possible candidate for such overall responsibility, had no powers to develop a policy, to control the services or to iron out deficiencies. If the services of 1939 needed anything it is clear that they needed an administrative overhaul.

For the patient a comprehensive service existed only for those who could pay, and those who could satisfy the means test requirements of the voluntary hospitals. The services as a whole presented a hotchpotch of entitlements and disqualifications with the result that many had to go without medical care or without the appropriate medical care. Within the services grave deficiencies were emerging:

21

general practitioners claimed to be overworked, isolated from one another and from hospitals and badly distributed geographically, whilst voluntary hospitals were facing growing financial difficulties and as a whole hospitals were reported as suffering from three major defects—inadequate accommodation (a shortfall of about one-third in hospital beds was estimated) shortage and maldistribution of specialists and the lack of co-ordination among hospitals in each area (Hospital Surveys). Local government services were reported as showing 'very great variations in the adequacy and efficiency of the services provided' (Wilson 1946); particularly among their hospital provisions. All in all the situation was far from satisfactory for administrator, doctor and patient alike.

Moves for change

Pressures for change there had always been, but it took the war and three particular events during it to precipitate the decision to create a National Health Service. The first of these was the creation and operation of the Emergency Medical Service (Titmus 1950) which, *inter alia*, brought the specialists out of their well-provided metropolitan and teaching hospitals and into contact with the average local hospital which was often small and very poorly equipped. Their reactions of horror were reflected in the many letters to the medical press at this time and is no doubt one of the factors behind the decision of Ernest Brown, the Minister of Health of the war-time coalition government in 1941 to set up, after the war, a comprehensive hospital service available for all making use of both voluntary and local government hospitals. He also announced that a survey of hospital facilities would be undertaken (Hospital Surveys).

At about the same time the Government had set up a small inter-departmental committee 'to undertake . . . a

22

survey of the existing national scheme of social insurance
and allied services . . .' (Beveridge 1942). The report of
this committee, the Beveridge Report, turned out to be a
war-time best seller and the foundation of much of the
social security legislation of the immediate post-war
period. Relevant to our purpose, the Report made it clear
that among the necessary pre-requisites of a social security
system was the establishment of 'a national health service',
a fact which was later to cause doctors to wonder if their
main task was to be government inspectors controlling the
use made of sickness and similar insurance benefits. (It
will be appreciated that any entitlement to sickness
benefits must depend, primarily, on a doctor's certification
of the claimant's illness.)

The proposal for a National Health Service was accepted
by the Government: it would be comprehensive of all
forms of treatment and cover all people. Sir John Ander-
son, the Government's spokesman, said that the Government envisaged co-operation between public and voluntary
authorities 'but public health must be someone's responsibility. Experience justified putting this ultimate responsibility in any area on the well-tried local government
machinery working very often over larger areas'. Private
practice would remain, voluntary hospitals would be safe-
guarded and the patient would retain the right to choose
his doctor. 'Negotiations' with interested bodies would
begin at once but, as his colleague the Chancellor of the
Exchequer, Sir Kingsley Wood said later in the Commons
debate, 'negotiations with the medical profession would
take a considerable time for it was essential when one is
dealing with a great honourable profession such as the
medical profession, that the matters that have to be settled
between it and the Government should be settled by
negotiation and achieved with the utmost amount of
goodwill'. 'Negotiations' or 'consultations', to use the word

23

that Herbert Morrison and Aneurin Bevan both preferred, were to begin at once.

The timetable of the discussions

(a) The Brown Plan

The Minister of Health, given the remit to begin discussions with the many pressure groups known to have views on and interest in the outcome of his decisions, must presumably have some views on what he would like to achieve and it is more than likely that many of these views came from his officials. Such seems to be the case with the discussion on a National Health Service for Brown's first 'plan' presented in the earliest discussions in March 1943 hardly seems to be the brain child of a liberal national, as by political persuasion he was. Indeed the plan bears striking resemblances to plans produced earlier by the National Association of Local Government Officers and the Society of Medical Officers of Health. It must be remembered in this context that many of the medical officers of the Ministry including the then Chief, Sir John Charles, had come from local government service and presumably had had contact with one or both of these bodies. There is little doubt for this and other reasons that what is subsequently called the Brown Plan was really the officials' plan based on their first thoughts. The contents of this plan have never been published but it is possible to piece together something of its main points. It envisaged a unified health service, all the services being the responsibility of one administrative unit, based on a system of regional local government units or possibly joint authorities. The voluntary hospitals services would be 'utilized' although what this meant is not clear: it is clear, however, that it implied something less than complete nationalization and removal of ownership. General practitioners were, apparently, to

24

be full-time salaried servants within this administrative system. In a phrase this plan was the administrator's idea of the tidy administrative plan, all services under one body neatly unified without devious administrative complications.

Such was the reaction of the British Medical Association's representatives that the Minister was forced to put his plan 'in the discard', a phrase which was subsequently to cause anxious medical men to turn to their knowledge of card games to see how far, if at all, cards 'in the discard' could be brought back into play. For the rest of 1943, Brown (having discarded his own plan) floundered as he listened to the conflicting views of the pressure groups. His promised White Paper on a proposed plan gradually faded further and further away. At the end of the year, whether because of this failure or not, he gave way at the Ministry to Henry U. Willink. He was more successful and early in 1944 produced his first (and the first published) plan, the White Paper of February 1944.

(b) The White Paper

In this, the White Paper Plan, far more details had been written in although many were still missing: a study of the various plans over the four years from 1943 to 1946 shows clearly how despite the concessions, compromises, and changes of mind that went on, the process of gradually filling in the details continued, each plan adding something to the previous one. The White Paper gave central responsibility to the Minister of Health advised by an appointed Central Health Services Council (one report on the Brown Plan spoke of nominations to such a body, but probably because of civil service pressure, this was never repeated). The local organization of all the services would be based on joint local authority areas, the joint authorities being advised by local versions of the Central Health Services

Council. The authority would take over local authority hospitals and lay down the conditions under which voluntary hospitals would participate and, in return, they would receive grants towards part of the cost of patient care. General practitioner services would be related to the plans of the joint authorities in an unspecified way, but the doctors would be under contract to a central medical Board together with local committees. The doctor would be paid 'as in the National Health Insurance system' (Braithwaite 1957) on a *per capita* system unless he worked in a joint authority provided health centre when his remuneration would be by way of 'salary or similar alternative'. The central medical Board would have the power to refuse doctors the right to practise in certain areas, and, under certain conditions, to compel new doctors to work in poorly served areas.

(c) The Willink Plan

The process of change in the plans (or 'erosion' as Arthur Greenwood for the Opposition once called it) had begun as the Government sought to modify their views to meet those of the pressure groups, but as we shall see this first move away from the original Brown Plan failed to satisfy many of the groups. The White Paper invited discussion and these went on for some fifteen months (with a break in the summer of 1944 when travelling was forbidden or heavily restricted as the massing of troops and supplies for the D-Day landings on the coasts of Normandy reached their peak) by which time a revised plan, the Willink Plan, had been drawn up. Again it was not published but confidential versions of it went to the main groups and a close persual of their journals and other sources enables us to outline its proposals. Willink himself said in a later debate in the Commons on the National Health Service Bill that he had, by May 1945, reached such a stage in the discussion that he found it possible to begin drafting the necessary legislation.

The central administration in this Willink Plan represents no change in principle but rather a further building up of the detail: the membership of the Central Health Services Council was outlined and special standing advisory committees proposed to meet the need for specialized advice, all of which Bevan took over almost unaltered. Below the national level the attempt to meet the conflicting views on the local administration, brought forth a complicated solution. A two-tier system of planning bodies for all services was proposed, with, as the top tier, regional authorities based on medical teaching hospitals (forerunners of the Regional Hospital Boards of the service of today). The second tier would be area planning authorities equivalent in size to the joint authorities of the earlier plans. These area authorities would submit plans for all but hospital services to the regions and the plans would be binding on constituent bodies once they had been approved by the Minister. Hospital planning groups, made up of equal representation from local authority and voluntary hospitals and parallel to the area bodies, would do the same for the hospital plans which the regional bodies would marry with the other plans before submission to the Minister. Local authorities and voluntary hospital bodies would remain as executive units for their own hospitals.

For the general practitioners, the powers of direction for the Central Medical Board went and instead local committees were proposed on the lines of a modified version of the Insurance Committees of the National Health Insurance system—a proposal which was later to be accepted, in large part, by Bevan. The issue of remuneration was shelved for a committee to tackle, but without direction it was felt that financial inducements would be

27

needed to persuade doctors to go to the less fortunate areas. Health centres, a key feature of the White Paper, were relegated to an 'experimental' status and the right to sell the goodwill of medical practices, taken away in the White Paper, was reinstated. Willink was thus still trying to achieve some unification if only at the planning level while trying to meet as many points of view as possible.

(d) The National Health Service Bill

The end of the European war saw the end of the war-time coalition government, a general election and the return in high summer of the Labour Government with Aneurin Bevan as Minister of Health. As we shall see he introduced little that was new, the only major point being the nationalization of hospitals but he retraced some of the steps that Willink had taken, and for the rest, he took over much of the detail progressively worked out in pre-ceding plans. He had one new group to conciliate, his own political party, but for them, pledged in an earlier docu-ment to a full-time salaried service based on regional local government and very like the Brown Plan in many of its details, he made few concessions.

After his arrival at the Ministry he stayed silent for a long time and, on his own admission, did little 'negotia-tion'. He presented his Bill in March 1946 and it received the Royal Assent in virtually the same form in November of that year. The decisions on the framework had been taken and the pressure groups had played their part. The process was not however complete and negotiations or consultations went on up until the day the service began on July 5, 1948. By then however the discussions were about the lesser details, the major decisions having been embodied in the Act—this, however, is not to suggest that all was amity and light after 1946, there were many harsh words and threatening gestures to follow but these are in

28

a period beyond the confines of this study (Eckstein 1960).

(B) The pressure groups and their views

Popular imagery of pressure groups no doubt often conjures up thoughts of strong arm tactics, of threats and of a Government v. pressure group confrontation. The true position, however, in the National Health Service discussions was very different for it was important that the Ministry should learn something of the views of, and gain expertise from, those already responsible for elements of the health services. To have done otherwise was to risk (at worst) a sterile plan or at best one which was less efficient and workable than it might have been; pressure groups were, therefore, in this light a necessary part of the decision-making process. Not only was this part of the public image wrong, but the concept of a pressure group v. Government confrontation was also only partially true. As we shall see, on many issues the groups were in conflict one with another: e.g. the bitter discussion between the medical profession who were opposed to local government control in any shape or form and the local government associations who were anxious to keep their existing powers and if possible extend them. This particular area of decision-making, as with so many others in the National Health Service, involved a many-sided discussion and as such is probably a truer picture of the relationship between Government and pressure groups in all sorts of spheres of policy decisions.'

Space does not permit a semantic discussion on the term 'pressure group': suffice it to note that pressure groups are here taken as those organized groups who sought to influence the decisions the Government was taking. This is not to brand the groups as existing only or

29

mainly for this purpose; most, if not all, fulfilled many other roles of a more lasting kind, finding themselves temporarily, on this occasion, fulfilling the functions of a pressure group. In this study, the groups concerned can best be discussed by subdividing them into three categories —those with skills to offer, those with administrative machinery and know-how to offer and those with property to offer. In any league table of the successes achieved in the discussion, those with skills top the table and those with property fade to the bottom, especially after 1945 when faced by a Labour Government which was not so firmly wedded to property rights as to leave them undisturbed if other solutions were called for.

1 Pressure groups with skills to offer

First in any list of skilled groups in this context must come the medical profession, a profession which if united by common title, was not united organizationally. The main spokesman for the doctors was (and still is) the British Medical Association, representative of all types of medical work. In addition, there were the specialist organizations, the Royal Colleges representing consultant opinions, as well as the Society of Medical Officers of Health representing local government doctors, the Medical Practitioners Union, a doctors' Trade Union affiliated to the Trades Union Congress and the political medical bodies like the Socialist Medical Association. (Since the National Health Service came into being further medical organizations have been created, like for example, the College of General Practitioners and the Fellowship for Freedom in Medicine.) Realizing this division of the profession the Minister of Health, early in the discussions, asked for a joint representative committee which, with a British Medical Association majority, had representatives of most other medical organizations except what might be termed the trouble-some fringe, the Medical Practitioners Union and the Socialist Medical Association. It was this body that negoti-ated with the successive ministers of health and to which references hereafter to the medical profession as distinct to the British Medical Association apply.

The doctors were, of course, not the only profession to have discussions at the Ministry of Health. There were many others, which if we were to list them all would add little of value, but some will merit mention from time to time in the pages that follow. It should, perhaps, be added that on many of the issues the professions thought alike, but on others they were divided within themselves, between themselves and between themselves and the medical profession. The unity displayed was therefore sometimes more apparent than real; one reason for this was that the creation of the National Health Service seemed to offer opportunities for some groups, e.g. dentists, to throw off the shackles of medical control and become completely independent. The National Health Service too seemed to offer the perfect prospect for a race to the glories of full professional status, and some of the groups, as we shall see, tried to take the opportunities offered. Others like the dentists, physiotherapists and many more, had to wait until the Service was many years old before their professional aspirations were realized (Supplementary Professions).

2 Pressure groups of administrative organizations

In the second category of the groups representing adminis-trative organizations, several can be listed but none more important than the local government associations, i.e. asso-ciations of similar types of local authorities. The major pair were the County Councils Association representing

County Councils, and the Association of Municipal Corporations representing county and non-county boroughs. The smaller authorities were represented by the Rural District Councils Association and the Urban District Councils Association. United in defining what they had and in calling for the reform of local government whilst at the same time failing to agree on a reformed shape for local government, they were perhaps accorded more power than their divided condition tactically deserved. Also in this category of groups representing organizations were the National Association of Insurance Committees, representing the local committees of the National Health Insurance 'panel' system and the voluntary hospitals, although they perhaps fit more happily in the third category. Like the local authority associations both these groups tended to stand for the *status quo*, together with more responsibilities if that were possible.

3 Pressure groups with property at stake

Finally, the third category of groups representing property, has two groups, those local government associations whose members owned hospitals, and the voluntary hospital organization, the British Hospitals Association. Representing the medically powerful voluntary hospitals this latter group had considerable power whilst its property remained intact. It had, too, a great strength in the loyalty of the medical profession most, if not all, of whom had trained in voluntary hospitals and most of whom regarded the system as much superior to that of the local government hospitals. Once, however, they lost their property, their influence declined, although the peculiar contribution and features of the voluntary hospital still lives on into the second decade of the hospital service. Even if its architecture does not betray its ancestry, most experienced hospital visitors can still quickly spot an ex-voluntary hospital from an ex-local authority hospital.

The reader of many of the journals and articles of the period will perhaps be surprised to discover no organized group representing the user or potential user of the service: the only spokesmen for both the paymaster and the public was Parliament and the Government. How far and in what directions they can lay claims to have protected the public interest is hard to say. That there is a service, that it is available at little or no direct cost, that all can use it if they wish, these presumably are successes enough: for the rest, the organization of the service is a technicality on which the public had few if any views and certainly no organized institution to put them forward. The public was presumably only interested in the result: the groups did from time to time lay claim to seeking to promote the public welfare more often than not, it seems, to act as a cover or justification for their own self-interests. There is, therefore, some truth in the claim that the only person not represented round the Minister's table was the patient.

The views of the groups prior to the first round of discussions

As we have suggested the reform of the health services had been in the air for some time before 1942 so it is somewhat surprising to discover that for many of the groups, viewpoints were only formed (or perhaps published) after the discussions at the Ministry of Health started. For the rest it makes a useful starting point for the rest of this book to see where they all stood on some of the health service issues just before the discussions began.

On the basic question of the need for reform and overhaul of the services and the development of a comprehensive health service, most groups seemed to be in favour.

33

This general favour bestowed on the broad idea however covered a considerable measure of disagreement on the methods of achieving such a service. In general terms the political organizations of the left favoured a service which was fully available to all irrespective of income; i.e. they wanted a total population coverage. In opposition to them were groups like the British Medical Association, the National Association of Insurance Committees and others who favoured what came to be known as the 90% proposal. This said that the service should be extended to workers not at that time covered by the 'panel' system but of a similar status and income level as the existing beneficiaries, and to all their dependants; this, it was estimated, would cover about 90% of the population who would have a free comprehensive health service, leaving the richest tenth of the population to buy their own medical care, thus protecting the existence of private medical services.

There were two solutions, at this time, being canvassed to the problem of the central administration of the National Health Service: one favoured by the professions, something on the lines of a public corporation divorced from day to day political control and largely under the control of fellow professionals. The other view, more often assumed rather than stated, was for the normal system of a Governmental department subject to Parliamentary control. Both views agreed that the central body should exclusively deal with all health services, an almost unanimous view which was never conceded at this time by the Government. The Ministry of Health in fact, remained responsible for housing services for several years after the Act was passed, and even today is still not responsible for many health services, the school medical service, for example.

On the more detailed matters of administration less is

known of the views of the groups, probably because many had not seriously considered such topics. For the hospital service of the future, most groups with any views at all made some reference to regional control or planning, although the British Medical Association (and probably other professional groups too) always added the rider that the regionalism must not be a regional system of local government. The co-operation of voluntary and local authority hospitals gained unanimous, and indeed inevitable, agreement with few if any references to nationalization. On the general practitioner services, controversy before 1943 centred on three points. The first was the administrative control of the service, with the medical and other professions being opposed and the local authority associations in favour of local government control; no other alternatives were canvassed until later in the discussions. The remuneration of general practitioners was a second bone of contention: the British Medical Association favoured *per capita* payments whilst local government and politically leftish organizations favoured a full-time salaried service. It was on this point that the bitterest of discussions centred as successive Ministers tried to change the methods of remuneration: it is a subject on which the doctors and the Ministry have rarely seen eye to eye leading in 1949, to an amending Act, (Act 1949) to a Judicial Review in the early 1950s, to a Royal Commission later in the same decade (Royal Commission 1960) and finally to the current (1965) situation where the system of remuneration once so ardently desired by the profession now seems unacceptable. Remuneration has come to be one of the most troublesome words in the National Health Service (Eckstein 1960). Finally the third trouble spot in the general practitioners' service on which some pre-1943 views are available was the 'health centre', its role, the need for it and its provision and control.

35

On the future of local government health services such views as there were either took the professional standpoint of removing as much as possible from local government (the Society of Medical Officers of Health, of course, disagreeing) or concentrating on the more generic arguments about the reform of the system of local government —i.e. what are the services that ought to be locally controlled and by which sort of local authority?

Paying for the proposed services was rarely mentioned, Beveridge's proposals for a combination of National Insurance contributions, rates and taxes attracting little comment. Most groups, and especially the professions, accepted the patient's right to choose his doctor, and to opt for private practice if he so desired. There was less unanimity, especially from the groups of the political left, for the idea of the doctor's being able to provide both public and private treatment.

These were the views of a few of the more important groups, and for the rest, views began to form as the implications of the creation of a National Health Service became recognized. These views are briefly set out because in many cases their expression had been vague and generalized. But the seeds of the future disagreements were already apparent: how they came to the surface and the progress of the Whitehall discussions is the subject of the succeeding chapters of this book.

3

The financing of the service
and the population to be covered

In this and the succeeding chapters the National Health
Service is subdivided into sections and the course of discussions and the build up of the final form of each section
in turn is set out. Each chapter outlines the main alternative solutions available and traces the choices made from
one plan to the next. It is unlikely that the sectionalism
adopted here was in the minds of the various ministers as
they were taking decisions: it is rather a methodology
for ordering the data we present. In this chapter, as a
basic starting point, we concern ourselves with three
general topics, the general reaction to the service, its
financing and its population coverage: each is taken in
turn.

(A) General reactions to the various plans

As will be seen, it is not always easy to disentangle the
general reactions of the groups to the various plans—they
tended, naturally enough, to be strongly influenced by the
parts of the plans most relevant to their own situation.
Nonetheless the general tenor of some of their reactions

are worth setting out if only to get the general climate of response.

(a) The Brown Plan

We begin with the Brown Plan early in 1943 which had only a short and very unhappy life. Alone among the medical groups, the Socialist Medical Association welcomed the plans as something approximating to their views of a unified, socialized medical service and in a sense this welcome to the plan was the kiss of death for most of their medical colleagues. The British Medical Association, on the other hand, claimed it to be, in one of their milder phrases, an 'unfruitful basis for discussion'. Their spokesman, Dr. Charles Hill suggested that the Government was hurrying forward with this part of the Beveridge Report alone because it wanted to control the medical profession, and through it, the issue of medical certificates upon which any payments for sickness benefits would be made. At this stage the British Medical Association's Council made two pre-conditions to its co-operation in preparing a National Health Service; firstly that 'the character, terms and conditions of the medical service (be) determined by negotiation and agreement with the medical profession' and secondly that provision be made for those not wanting to avail themselves of the service and preferring private medical care. Of the other medical organizations who mainly agreed with the Association's view, one can quote the Medical Practitioners' Union which felt that it could not trust the Minister and its members saw themselves as 'fighting tooth and nail for (their) liberties in the national sphere'. Such views are enough to emphasize that the negotiations had got off to a bad start from the medical point of view.

On what might almost be termed the other side of the fence, the local government associations made little reference to this plan beyond the comment that the reform of local government itself should precede any reform of its services. This was a position they were to cling to despite their manifest inability to agree among themselves on a suitable basis for such a reform of local government. Central government was, however, right, in all the circumstances, in not wanting to grasp the nettle of local government reform at the expense of delaying service reforms highly desired by the general public. To have frustrated the general enthusiasm for social reform might well have had a serious effect on the morale of civilian and serviceman alike. In local government circles, therefore as in medical circles, little welcome was expressed for this first plan.

(b) The White Paper

There were few groups therefore to mourn the early demise of the Brown Plan or, one suspects, his departure from office. Better things were hoped for from his successor and his White Paper (White Paper 1944). At first the medical reactions were not hostile, the Socialist Medical Association's welcoming what it called a 'pivotal point in the history of British medicine' whilst the British Medical Journal found some temporary relief in it but claimed, nonetheless, to see a Government whose aim was to move towards a full-time salaried local government service. Of all the early medical comments on the White Paper, perhaps the neatest was that of *The Lancet* when it claimed that the White Paper 'approaches the millenium somewhat indirectly'.

The first medical reaction then was cautious and little happened whilst the democratic machinery of the British Medical Association ground out its views, a process made much longer by the Government's ban on travel during the summer of 1944 as the D-Day effort was built up and launched. When at last the Association set itself, along with other medical organizations, for the negotiations, its Chairman, Dr. H. G. Dain was able to say, 'We have expressed ourselves in favour of the development of the service. We have disapproved of the White Paper as it stands. . . . We prefer these services to proceed by evolution. . . . We have stated emphatically that we do not wish to be employed by local authorities, that there should be no civil direction, that there should be no whole-time salaried service for general practice and that we shall have no clinical control.' As *The Times* put it the next day: 'from an impressive mass of negative resolutions it emerges only that the conference has willed almost all the ends and rejected almost all the means'. All the doctors wanted, the leader writer thought, was to be left alone and, in the compass of a sentence or two, this is a fair comment on the negative attitude of the Association at this time. Despite obvious improvements over the Brown Plan from their point of view (e.g. the disappearance of full-time salaried service, local government control, etc.) they were still far from satisfied.

The local authority associations were meantime still protesting that local government reform must be put first or, if not, that the proposed changes in local authority duties must be regarded as temporary pending such a reform. They were still hardly taking the matter seriously despite 'long and arduous discussions': rather they were hoping against hope for local government reform.

Speaking for the voluntary hospitals, the British Hospitals Association welcomed the aims of the White Paper and were relieved to find their continued existence was included, but they felt that the proposals of the plan, especially on the financing of their services, might eventually lead to their extinction. Elsewhere among the remaining groups, despite the occasional tongue in the cheek, the

White Paper was widely welcomed, and this first public plan served to rally support among the many less deeply involved groups, some of whom were to look on later 'concessions' with alarm. On the whole, the medical profession and voluntary hospitals excepted, the Minister had done far better than perhaps he had the right to hope for.

(c) The Willink Plan

The Willink Plan of 1945 was, as we have seen, a confidential plan and public comment is therefore somewhat scarce. By now, it was the turn of the politically left groups to express alarm. The Socialist Medical Association spoke of the 'White Paper in danger', the Trades Union Congress called on the Minister to stand firm and the Labour Party regretted the Minister's contemplation of radical alterations in the scheme 'violating democratic principles and sacrificing the health of the people to the vested interests of the medical profession'. The boot was now firmly on the other foot, and although not completely satisfied with some of the details, as we shall see, the major medical organizations were much happier. Local government, too, seemed reasonably happy for, as they told a Select Committee of the House of Commons much later, their preference was for the Willink Plan rather than the Act of 1946. Willink had got to the point therefore where some of the major groups were feeling reasonably content and only the vociferous but not apparently very powerful bodies of the political left were complaining.

(d) The National Health Service Bill

Then came the change of Government and another Minister. His silence for several months worried the medical profession and their request for a meeting was met with the response that he was willing to do so as soon as he was

THE FINANCING OF THE SERVICE

ready. In the interim therefore, the profession's joint negotiating committee felt the need to state its point of view in seven principles. These principles which were dismissed by the Medical Practitioners Union as 'seven futile clauses' and the Socialist Association as 'completely unprincipled' are worthy of summary. The first stated opposition to a full-time salaried service in government or local government hands. The second spoke of professional freedom, the third of the patient's right to choose his doctor and to choose private treatment if he so desired. The fourth claimed the doctor's right to choose where he would work and the fifth his right to participate in the service. The sixth spoke of hospitals planned over 'natural hospital areas centred on universities in order that these centres of education and research may influence the whole service' and the final one called for adequate medical representation on all the administrative bodies of the service 'in order that doctors may make their contribution to the efficiency of the service'. In this way, the medical profession drew the line on which they were prepared to do battle.

Armed with these principles they met the Minister who, they complained, 'listened' but did not 'negotiate'. These meetings early in 1946 preceded the publication of the Bill and its subsequent passage through Parliament. At first their reactions were apprehensive rather than condemnatory, but eventually the British Medical Association found the Bill unacceptable on the grounds of its control over areas in which a doctor could practise, the state ownership of hospitals and doubts over the methods of remuneration. Once the Bill had become law medical tempers rose and opposition stiffened to a showdown in 1948, an event outside the time span of this study. During the passage of the Bill however the profession's main spokesmen were surprisingly quiet; but perhaps it will not seem surprising

42

when, in a final chapter, we draw up a balance sheet of successes.

The 'troublesome' medical groups were divided on the Bill—the Medical Practitioners Union found it 'disappointing from the point of view of the general practitioner', whilst the Socialist Medical Association was once again happy despite the exclusion of its own major aims for the service.

Meanwhile the dentists were patting themselves on the back for what they claimed was their part in the development of full dental services, but through their journal, the *British Dental Journal* they were claiming that the Bill showed little evidence of the Government understanding the special problems of dentistry.

While the local government organizations were bemoaning their loss of powers, the Labour Party was welcoming a Bill which looked little like its own original proposals (Labour Party 1943). The Conservative Party was critical of the methods seeming, naturally enough, to prefer the solutions of its own ex-minister. As the Conservatives did at no time, as far as can be discovered, produce a separate party proposal for a National Health Service, it is hardly surprising that they stuck to the Willink Plan. The opposition, though, was not whole-hearted and the whole level of political criticism seemed muted in favour of what was believed to be the general public welcome for the idea of a National Health Service. It seemed politically dangerous to be against the Service : no one under the force of public opinion questioned the fundamental decision and instead some tried the difficult task of accepting the aim but regretting the methods.

To sum up it can be said that the general reactions to the plans of the successive ministers for a National Health Service were always generally favourable and such opposition as there undoubtedly was became centred on some of the specific aspects to be discussed in later chapters. There was little or no overt opposition to the service *per se* so that Government and groups were working to an agreed end even if differing on methods.

(B) Financing the service and the population to be covered

It is, of course, impossible to say how each minister approached his task but it is theoretically possible to conceive a process whereby under each element of the planning of the National Health Service the various available alternatives were examined, and one chosen, perhaps subsequently to be rejected under pressure or convincement. It, therefore, is necessary to begin with a brief statement of the alternative courses open to the Government.

On the issue of how many people should be covered by the service (and by this it seems to have been generally accepted that coverage meant the provision of a free comprehensive service), three alternatives were canvassed. The first, which never appealed to more than a few groups, was the idea of 100% coverage with no alternative private care, that is a monopolistic health service with no competitor. The second, which the Government adopted and never seriously considered altering, was that of 100% coverage with the alternative of private medical care available for those who wanted and could afford it. As we shall see there were two transient criticisms of this; one from the Labour Party insisting that those who opted out should not escape their share of the cost of the National Health Service, and the opposite viewpoint, canvassed at one stage by the British Medical Association, that those who opted out get a grant-in-aid from the Government in return for what they had paid for a service they did not use. The third alternative open to the Government was for something less than 100% coverage and theoretically many limits to the coverage could have been made, but the one that attracted the most support came to be called the 90% proposal. This implied extending the coverage afforded under National Health Insurance schemes to similarly placed people not previously covered and to all their dependants, a total of approximately 90% of the population. Although, as we shall see, this view got some support, mainly from the medical profession, it does not appear to have held any attraction for the successive ministers each committed to the Beveridge proposals of 100% coverage.

The financing of the service offered innumerable alternatives including a range from the patient bearing the total cost through to the national exchequer bearing all the cost. Except that the decision to remove the cost from the patient seemed a necessary and acceptable part of the service to all (or most) taking part in the discussions, the exact ways of raising the money would depend, in large measure, on decisions on the administrative structure of the service.

Public reactions to the Brown proposals were few, although the British Medical Association did hesitantly accept the Beveridge proposals of 100% coverage but recalled the recommendation of their Medical Planning Commission in 1942 for the 'evolution' of the service, in this terminology, the 90% coverage. As the *British Medical Journal* said, it 'would be undemocratic, not to say foolish, for the medical profession to run counter to the rest of the community at a time when it needs all its sympathy and support in what is the gist of the matter, namely the determination of the conditions and terms of service'. Before, however, the end of 1943, and the appearance of the next plan, the representative body of the British Medical Association at its annual meeting accepted a resolution which amounted to a variant on the 90% theme. The White Paper did not, however, weaken on this point; the services would be freely available to all, although with the right of those who so desired to buy private treatment outside the service. On financing, the White Paper took over the proposals of the Beveridge Report that a sum be set aside from National Insurance funds for the health services (without making contribution conditions as a necessary qualification for National Health Service care) and in total, its estimates of cost showed this amount to be 27% of the cost, the taxpayer paying 36·6% and the local ratepayer a further 36·4% (this, of course, was not the complete cost as voluntary hospitals would play some financial part in this service). In 1939 public expenditure on public medical service showed 20% from contributions, 6% from the taxpayer and 74% from the ratepayer. The proposals, therefore were for an increased burden to rest on the taxpayer, a burden which was seriously under estimated in amount and proportion when the service finally became operative.

Towards the end of the year the British Medical Association again expressed its preference for the 90% proposal, as did the National Association of Insurance Committees. The financial proposals on the other hand attracted little attention and those for the 100% coverage, with the two exceptions mentioned, seemed acceptable to most groups.

In the Willink Plan of 1945, the Government showed itself unwilling to concede the points made by the medical profession, which, according to the British Medical Journal, concluded that it would be 'illogical to try and exclude one tenth of the population' from the service. They were, however, still emphasizing the importance of private practice in maintaining the freedom of the doctor, for the man with other sources of income could never become the tool of Government. The representative body of the association, therefore, decided not to press for the 90% proposal but instead to tell the Minister that they were willing 'to negotiate terms and conditions for such a 100% service, if such be decided upon, provided that ample safeguards (were) introduced to ensure that any member of the community, whatever his income, should be enabled to obtain his medical services, in part or in whole, privately, as for example by grant-in-aid provisions'. Here was a bid to make private practice much wider and theoretically open to more than the top 10% of the population. Such a proposal, however, of allowing non-users to be compensated for their non-use of statutory services ran counter to traditional methods of financing statutory public services. In the subsequent general election neither political party expressed support for other than the 100% coverage with the parallel continuation of private practice for those who wanted to pay.

The publication of the National Health Service Bill changed little under any of the subject matter of this section, except that the disappearance of voluntary hospitals in their existing form robbed the service of the potential contributions of their finances. Standing virtually alone on its 90% proposals and supporting it in a way which could easily appear to the public as a selfish concern for its own financial interests, the medical profession was doomed to failure on this score. It seems clear, too, that despite public pronouncements a sizeable proportion of the membership of the British Medical Association was not opposed to the 100% coverage. The Council of the Association probably recognized that to force this issue might have risked a split in the ranks and, as we shall glimpse during the period of the study (and see more clearly if going beyond the Act), the profession was often fatally divided. Indeed Bevan was later to court, quite deliberately, the consultant and so split the professional opposition to his Act.

We may sum up this chapter by noting that the points discussed here were broad issues on which public and political party opinion seemed fairly clear and which did not, within the acceptance of a National Health Service, greatly affect individual groups. These groups, by their very nature, exist to serve sectional and specialized interests, and it is therefore to be expected that they concentrated less on these general aspects and more on the sections likely to affect those interests.

4

The central administration and the advisory machinery

It is theoretically possible to think of many alternative structures for the central administrative and advisory machinery of a service such as the National Health Service, but in practical terms the possibilities are much more limited. We can discuss these alternatives under three headings: the degree of central control, the type of central controlling body and the advisory machinery to that body.

The degree of central control can be taken to imply the relationships between central and local administrative units, but the exact power of one *vis-à-vis* the other is hard to define. It seems clear that, throughout the discussions, the aim of all the participants was to achieve as great a measure of executive decentralization as possible, with perhaps occasional overtones of some limited centralization in planning. In the main the choice seemed to be for control at the periphery rather than at the centre, the proposition never being seriously questioned. Also implied under this heading is the question of the services controlled. Whilst no one suggested that the armed forces medical services be under the control of that central body, most of the groups spoke of all civilian health services being unified under one control, including, for example, such services as the industrial medical services or the school medical services. At the same time they felt that the central body should be exclusively concerned with health services, a point which no minister was prepared to concede. One suspects that the political ministers saw limited opportunities of making a reputation in running the National Health Service and greater opportunities in some of their other responsibilities, particularly housing.

The second heading, the type of central body, presented more definite alternatives. Three main alternatives were canvassed, one supported, *inter alia*, by the Socialist Medical Association and the Society of Medical Officers of Health was for the traditional ministerial department whilst the second, supported by the British Medical Association among many others, was for a public corporation removed from the day to day political arena (the B.B.C. was often quoted as an example) to run the health services. The third proposal was a derivative of the second, including several corporations, each with responsibility for specific segments of the health services, a proposal favoured by the smaller professions who feared both political and medical domination. Their claim each time was that the special nature of their services was beyond the understanding of lay people.

Ministers at no time displayed any interest in any solution but the continuation of a ministerial department. The groups, however sadly, soon were to appreciate this and to concentrate their attention on a strong advisory machinery in which they had a powerful voice. The history that follows suggests that the groups had to wring concessions out of a department unwilling to concede any power to such machinery. It may be that the ministers felt their own professional staff competent to advise them and that these officials were jealous of any outside advice reaching the Minister. There was the example before the groups of the lack of success of the pre-war advisory machinery to make them wary of the Government's reaction to some of their proposals (Vernon 1940).

(a) The Brown Plan

The Brown Plan set the pattern for a central government department advised by some central body: a pattern which although altered in detail was never changed in major principle. According to a speech by Dr. Charles Hill, the British Medical Association spokesman, the central department was to be a basically reformed Ministry of Health. Its advisory body would be predominantly medical in membership, three quarters being nominated by the profession, and it would have the right to issue its own Reports. Here, if Dr. Hill was right, was the concept of a representative rather than an expert body. Nomination together with the right to issue reports was never again conceded by the ministers—to have done so was to run the risk of unacceptable advisers and advice.

The British Medical Association greeted this part of the plan with a plea for a corporate body (public corporation) going on to say that whatever was decided, agreement with the Minister on the administrative structure was a prerequisite to discussion on other things. The British Hospitals Association, too, spoke out through its Chairman, Sir Bernard Docker, for a Central Hospitals Board to advise on hospital services: they never wanted any executive body which could control their activities and therefore called only for an advisory body. The pharmacists called for a Pharmacy Commission composed of doctors and pharmacists under the Ministry of Health to ensure an adequate service for all controlling the entrance of new pharmacists to areas already well provided with pharmacists. This latter point is an interesting contrast with later medical objections to such a control, but in the case of the pharmacists they had their reasons. Their claim for full professional status was, they felt, handicapped by their members having to sell cosmetics and the like to make a living. They hoped to achieve such a position in which they worked full-time as pharmacists without the shopkeeper trappings, and hence the need for control and restriction.

(b) The White Paper

These calls for separate bodies were the forerunners of many later claims for separate professional administrations but to have conceded them all (or any of them) would have made a mockery of the power of any one central organization like the Ministry of Health. The White Paper of 1944 therefore confirmed the choice of central body, the Ministry of Health responsible in the traditional way to Parliament. The Minister would be advised in his health service duties by a Central Health Services Council which whilst primarily medical in composition would include representatives of the hospitals and of the other professions concerned. It would be appointed by the Minister, would advise and initiate advice, but the Minister would report annually to Parliament on its work. It would have the right to appoint specialized sub-committees and co-opt thereto, but all advice would come from and in the name of the Council with its medical majority. This advisory machinery was then to be expert rather than representative and would not have the same powers alleged to have been offered in the first plan.

The Council of the British Medical Association at once criticized the continued dispersal of health responsibilities throughout many Ministries and the continued responsibility of the Ministry of Health for such controversial matters as housing. The advisory machinery, too, proved unacceptable to them. Instead they proposed a central body exclusively responsible for all civilian health services advised by a body predominantly medical in composition, whose members would be elected. All the regulations made under the Act should have to be submitted by the Ministry to this advisory body before becoming operative. (This marks an interesting parallel with the powers of the National Insurance Advisory Committee under the National Insurance Acts which has a power similar to this). The proposed advisory body would initiate advice, publish its own reports and have an independent secretariat. The power to publish its own reports and have an independent secretariat was felt to be a safeguard against Ministry suppression and domination. Here was a clear statement of the demand for a powerful and independent advisory system, one form of protection against the lay control the profession so much feared.

One by one the various medical organizations came to agree with the British Medical Association on the primary importance of getting the 'right' administrative structure and hence a lot of medical effort was devoted in the subsequent discussions to that end. In the meantime the local government organizations were thinking only of local government reform and had little to say on this aspect of the White Paper.

Among many of the other groups the demands for specialized units of administration grew after the appearance of the White Paper. The British Hospitals Association reiterated its claim for a Central Hospitals Advisory Body with power to publish its own reports. The dental profession wanted election to the Central Health Services Council and the establishment of a separate central dental Board composed mainly of dentists. Unlike the hospitals, they wished their central body to have executive powers. The Royal College of Nursing called for a separate advisory council on nursing and midwifery with representation on the Central Health Services Council. Interestingly they were one of the few organizations not to call for the election of representatives on the advisory bodies. The College felt that not only did election not necessarily secure the best person for the job, but also that as most members of the profession at any point in time are student or assistant nurses, then most of the profession's elected representatives would be of this level.

The pharmacists wanted a central pharmacy Board with powers of control and the opticians wanted a central optical Board, the latter using reasons similar to those outlined earlier and used by the pharmacists. If the repetition bores, at least the point is underlined again and again, that each professional group wanted separate administrative structures, (sometimes executive, sometimes advisory) to meet the special problem of their individual services.

(c) On the Willink Plan

As a result of the long discussions that went on this point, the next plan, the Willink Plan, whilst leaving untouched the proposals concerning the Ministry of Health, recast somewhat the advisory machinery. The Minister was to be advised by a statutory body, the Central Health Services Council whose duty it would be to provide and initiate expert advice. It would be appointed and be representative of the main professional viewpoints, but with a medical majority. (The 37 proposed members included 19 doctors (including 6 ex-officio from certain medical organizations) 5 from voluntary hospitals, 5 from local authority hospitals, 2 nurses, 3 dentists, 1 midwife and 2 pharmacists. The Act of 1946 merely added another group, 2 lay and 2 medical representatives of the mental health services, turned the voluntary hospital representatives into hospital representatives and left the rest unchanged.) To assist the council, there would be Standing Advisory Committees (2 laid down by statute for medicine and hospitals and the remainder to be settled between the Minister and the council) whose specialist advice would go to the council and to the Minister to whom they would have direct access. The council would, however, have the right to ask the Minister to hold up action on any advice from a Standing Advisory Committee until it had commented upon it. The members of the council and Standing Advisory Committees would be appointed after consultations and the council would be free to elect its chairman and to appoint one of two joint secretaries. The Minister would be required to consult the council in framing all the regulations under the Act and he would be bound to publish the annual reports of the council unless it were not in the public interest to do so.

Here were major 'concessions' to the groups. The machinery had become stronger, the demands for separate professional advisory bodies had in part been met and the balance between the overall medical control through its majority on the council and the individual professions had been moved somewhat in latter's favour. Although the medical profession, therefore, had grounds for some pleasure, this loosening of their control was not to their liking.

A move at a special meeting in May 1945 of the British Medical Association's Representative Body to insist on a public corporation was successfully resisted by the Chairman on the grounds that the medical profession was in a much stronger position with the Minister than it would be in relation to the 'five medical despots', a reference to the corporation idea. The medical profession, at that time, always seemed (and still is) ambivalent about the necessary evils of control: if the control is lay, they will not understand the problems of medical services, but if they are medical, then they may understand too much. The Association's meeting went on to ask its negotiators to seek amendments designed to strengthen the power of the Central Health Services Council with its medical majority over the Standing Advisory Committee, thus showing that Willink had, in medical eyes, gone too far in his concessions to the 'other side'. Although a small example, this is an illuminating glimpse of how delicate the point of balance between conflicting views that the Minister was seeking.

Dentists seemed happy enough but asked for more seats on the council. The pharmacists too wanted more seats, although they were warned by their secretary that they could hope for little more: 'it seemed natural to balance pharmacists with dentists'. One wonders why? The Trades Union Congress, on the other hand wanted both more seats for 'health workers' and fewer seats for doctors. But when all is said, the point of balance was just about reached by Willink, as the formula in the Act itself reveals.

(d) The National Health Service Bill

The National Health Service Bill adopted most of the proposals in the Willink Plan—the only major changes being the dropping of the interesting power of the Central Health Services Council to review regulations, and the omission of any statutorily defined Standing Advisory Committees. An examination of the appropriate sections of the Act will thus soon show how the discussions of earlier ministers played a part in the final product.

The British Medical Association, on the publication of the Bill, sought to strengthen the Council's power over the Standing Advisory Committees and to gain a veto over appointments to the council. In neither case were they successful, although they must have felt some satisfaction at their achievements over the years on this part of the service.

Many of the other professions made attempts to secure professional administrations or at a second best, increased representation on the council. In Parliament, Bevan resisted all but one attempt to alter the balance of representation on the council begging his listeners not to allow an 'auctioning of seats on this Council'. The one successful amendment from the Opposition made it clear that the local authority and hospital representatives on the council must not be doctors, thus preventing any back door increase in the medical majority. Bevan took his main stand on the point of balance so painstakingly achieved by Willink. Asked to explain his distribution of seats, Bevan gave two clues to the reasoning behind the final solution. Speaking of the doctors' majority he said 'considering the doctor in the abstract, he is the person who, in himself, sums up all the various health services and therefore he has a different relationship to the health services as a whole'. On another occasion he defended the decision to have three dentists on executive councils and only two pharmacists, saying 'we are more short of dentists than we are of pharmacists'. Such, perhaps, were the reasons at the council level as well, and of such, in part at least is the stuff of power—scarcity value.

To sum up, the central body controlling the service was decided early on and the almost united opposition of the groups made no impact whatsoever. Here the groups were treading on very tender corns, the vested interests of politician and civil servant alike. Its degree of control was assumed rather than stated and this remained the position in the Act. It was on the outlet for frustrated administrative plans, the advisory machinery, that most of the discussion centred. In this area we can see the process of seeking an agreeable solution and the filling in of detail going on hand in hand and despite political party. Was all this effort worthwhile and has the advisory machinery achieved anything? A study of the operation of the service since 1948 would probably reveal that the importance of the advisory machinery was over-rated, perhaps because the Ministry has made little attempt to use any powers it may have to compel advice to be acted upon by the executive peripheral bodies.

5

Hospital and specialist services

In this chapter, the gradual building up of plans for the hospital services is discussed. In such a study as this only limited reference can be made to earlier discussion on the hospital services. These had been going on almost without a break since World War I and in the early months of World War II the complaints of consultants about the conditions of the hospitals mingled with discussions on possible reforms. Among the many that were suggested, one can single out the plan of Dr. Stephen Taylor (later Lord Taylor) for a regionally administered hospital service of nationally owned hospitals, almost, in fact, a blue-print for the solution of the National Health Service Act (Abel-Smith 1964). Although this plan and others attracted considerable attention in the columns of the medical press, they made little public impression and seemed to effect little the attitudes of the leaders of the medical profession. Clearly, the early war years saw a foment of ideas, but with surprisingly little impact. For a fuller account of this seminal period, a more lengthy history of hospitals than is possible here is needed (Abel-Smith 1964).

We have already noted the weaknesses of the 1939

59

services, the exclusion of hospital care from National Health Insurance benefits, the shortage of beds, of staff and the lack of co-ordination, and have hinted at how the creation of the war-time Emergency Medical Service threw many of these into high relief. Shortages could not be remedied by legislative means, but reorganization and availability could be, as indeed Brown recognized in his undertaking in 1941 to introduce a national hospital service at the end of the war. To do this, either separately or as part of a national health reform, the first administrative problem to be faced was whether to aim for a co-ordinated or a unified hospital service, i.e. dual ownership or some unification of ownership. Few voices, other than that of Dr. Taylor, spoke up in the political forum for the latter until the war was ending, and the major problem therefore became how to achieve co-ordination between voluntary and local authority hospitals to such an extent as to ensure adequate provision of all types of treatment without wasteful duplication. There was also the question, which in the end went unsolved, of how to relate the administration of the hospital services to those of the other health services; the ideal of administrative unification of all health services progressively gave way to separate administrative provisions for separate sections of the service.

The practical issue of co-ordination between voluntary and local authority hospitals turned on the composition, powers and financing of the co-ordinating bodies. Was the composition of this joint body to be equal representation irrespective of provision or was it to be related to the number of beds provided by each? Were its powers to be executive, thus diminishing if not actually removing the right of hospital ownership, or was it to be a planning body with the right to enforce its wishes or merely an advisory body? Given that government money would have to be fed into the system somewhere, would the joint body get the money and pass it on either on a bed or work done basis (during the war voluntary hospitals had done well on the bed grants often merely by keeping beds empty but available) (Abel-Smith 1964, Titmus 1950) or was the money to go directly to the hospital authorities?

A second major problem facing the Government, whether unifying or co-ordinating, was to decide on the area of the local unit of administration. There were those, including Dr. Taylor as already noted, who favoured regional authorities of some kind. The Nuffield Provincial Hospitals Trust had been created to promote the idea of regionalism which already had a favourable reception in medical circles, partly, no doubt, on the grounds of lessening or removing local authority power in the hospital world. There were those who spoke of somewhat smaller areas and yet others, including naturally enough the local government association, who thought in terms of existing local government boundaries.

At no stage in the discussion was the right of free treatment contested (except in so far as debate developed on the population to be covered) and as such the Government had, therefore, to find some means of ensuring that such treatment would be available as and when required.

(a) The Brown Plan

Little is known about the detail of the plan for this service. Brown talked of joint health boards to run all health services and he acknowledged them to be temporary expedients pending the reform of local government. He publicly said that the Government was looking to local government to take up this new duty, with some niche being found for the continued contribution of the voluntary hospitals. The reactions to this plan were rather more the reaction of groups jolted into thinking out (or restating) their viewpoints rather than specific answers to specific proposals.

The medical professions' leaders, at this point in time, were too incensed over the proposed local government salaried service to say much about hospitals. For the local authorities, however, the proposals of this part of the Brown Plan were getting very near home and they began to prepare their case. After the customary resolution calling for the prior reform of local government, the County Councils Association admitted that it was prepared to accept joint authorities, subject to safeguards, in cases of proved need. Their urban counterpart, the Association of Municipal Corporations, merely contented themselves with a call for local government reform.

Speaking in July of that year, on behalf of the British Hospitals Association, Sir Bernard Docker claimed that, in the public interest (almost a necessary clause in any pressure group claim) voluntary hospitals should be preserved as an essential factor in the nation's health and hospital services. Individual hospitals must retain considerable freedom and to that end, the methods of control and financing were of crucial importance. Voluntary hospitals must be enabled to take their proper share in the formulation of policy at the local level. These were, in a sense, warning shots from the Association of trouble ahead for the Minister.

At this time, too, the Labour Party went on record with their proposals (Labour Party 1943). They spoke of a unified health administration under democratically elected regional authorities. Voluntary hospitals would 'be brought into the national scheme on terms which will satisfy the nation's sense of equity'. In return for financial assistance, they would have to accept local authority representatives on their governing bodies. 'The effect of this scheme (would) be to ensure that before long the voluntary hospitals (would) come under the control of local authorities' so achieving a unified system. To an extent one can claim that the seeds of this section of the National Health Service Act lie here, but a closer look suggests that the claim of this document to the parentage of the Act is less than one might expect in an Act passed by a Labour Government.

The Brown Plan started groups thinking or, perhaps more correctly, putting their ideas on paper. Its attempts to achieve the unification of hospital and other health services was gradually whittled down and in each subsequent plan the need for hospitals to refer to other health services is diminished.

(b) The White Paper

The White Paper of 1944, as we have noted in other contexts, moved towards the views of some groups at the same time as it added more detail to the plan. The hospitals would be the responsibility of joint authorities advised by local versions of the Central Health Services Council. The joint authorities would take over and run all local authority hospitals whilst the voluntary hospitals that were willing to participate in the scheme would have to accept the area plan to be drawn up by the joint authority. These hospitals would be subject to inspection, but day to day control would be left to the voluntary hospitals' governing bodies. The grants that they would receive from the joint authorities would represent only part of the cost of the services provided, for, the White Paper argued, if all the costs were met, the voluntary income upon which the hospitals depended for their autonomy would dry up. This was the first detailed attempt to be made to achieve a marriage of what was probably two incompatibles—the independence of the voluntary hospitals and a co-ordinated hospital service.

One feature of the White Paper that received welcome from all medical and hospital groups except the Socialist Medical Association was the continuation of the dual hospital system of voluntary and local authority hospitals. The British Medical Association was far from happy, however, at the hospital proposals which they felt would lead to the gradual submersion of the voluntary hospital. 'These proposals would appear to illustrate once more the urge to control even a form of voluntary organization which, while uncontrolled, has achieved a magnificent standard of service to the community'. The Council of the Association proposed instead regional areas for hospital and medical services, the regional bodies to consist of representatives appointed by local authorities, the medical profession and the voluntary hospitals and their functions to be the planning of schemes and the disbursement of central monies. The medical profession had long favoured regionalization of the hospital services, and the final solution of regional hospital Boards owes a lot to their insistence on regional administration or planning; for the time being local authorities should continue to administer their own hospitals under the regional plan but each local authority should be compelled to have medical advisory committees with representation on the authorities' health committees. Once again the intense dislike of local government and its control of part of the hospital system was shown, a dislike which was an integral part of the medical profession's views on much of the National Health Service. The voluntary hospitals, the Association claimed, should be enabled to maintain and extend their services. Thus, in this way, the British Medical Association took the opportunity to make three of its longstanding viewpoints: regional planning, reduction of the local authorities' part in hospital services and the maintenance of the voluntary hospitals in which, of course, all doctors had had their training, and to whom many of the specialists owed their individual prestige and through that their lucrative private practices.

With the proposals of the white paper, the National Health Service plans were beginning to attack the very foundation of local government work in the hospital services. The County Councils Association's first response was therefore surprisingly mild when it called for more local authority control over the joint authorities and insisted that the bed grants to voluntary hospitals come only from the joint authorities instead of directly from the Government as some groups were proposing. They wanted to keep a major share of the responsibility in local government hands, a view which clashed directly with that of the medical profession. The Association of Municipal Corporations went a step further in wanting the joint authorities to be limited to planning on the grounds that other health services with which hospitals should be co-ordinated, would remain in local authority hands.

Later in the same year, 1944, the County Councils Association changed tack and came into line with the Association of Municipal Corporations calling for the proposed joint authorities' powers to be limited to planning. Administration involved the spending of public money which should only be done by local authorities, the elected representatives of the people. Voluntary hospitals accepting money from the joint authorities should have to accept public representation on their governing bodies and those not joining in the scheme should not be allowed to sabotage the joint authorities' plans by competitive extensions. If the voluntary hospitals were opposed to local government, the local authorities were equally jealous of the voluntary hospitals whose prestige and apparent success they always resented.

After a long discussion with the Minister, the appropriate committees of the council of the County Councils Association changed course again; they abandoned their claim for local authority administration of local government hospitals but instead asked for the creation of regional planning authorities (some twelve or thirteen in all) to be put above the joint administering authorities. Their full report bears striking similarities to the proposals that eventually came to be part of the Willink proposals of 1945, but because of travelling difficulties and because of yet more discussions at the Ministry, these committee reports were never accepted by the County Councils Association as its approved policy. It is, nonetheless, an interesting flirtation with the ideas of regionalism which so often in the past and for other purposes had been anathema to local government in general. However we may conclude that ideas were beginning to change in local government circles and that, like the Minister, they were facing the facts of the situation and leaving dogmatism in the search for practical solutions.

Meantime the British Hospitals Association, for the voluntary hospitals, rejected the White Paper's proposed joint authorities on the grounds that these administrative proposals did not afford the opportunity for the true partnership of voluntary and local authority that was essential for an efficient service. They also claimed that the financial proposals were inconsistent and unacceptable in affording only part payment for services rendered thus leaving the gap to be filled by voluntary income, whilst at the same time offering a free service and thereby discouraging the incentive to contribute to the voluntary hospitals. The proposal that the joint authorities administer the local authority hospitals directly was, strangely enough, objected to on the grounds that this would lead the authorities to favour their own hospitals at the expense of the voluntary hospitals. They wanted, they said, true partnership, free co-operation and co-ordination.

By the end of 1944 they were repeating their objections to the White Paper but interestingly had added to their counter proposals the suggestion of regional planning bodies. At about the same time the King Edward's Hospital Fund for London, came out with proposals for regional authorities—some twelve or thirteen in all—equally representative of local authority and voluntary hospitals. Like the local authorities, regionalism of some kind was gaining ground as a result of the discussion at the Ministry and when, in 1945, the details of the Willink Plan were circulated, it was clear that the Ministry, too, was moving towards regional solutions.

(c) The Willink Plan

Not only did Willink try to meet or succeed in convincing the groups on the merits of regionalism, but he went some long way to concede the views of local government. The joint authorities of the White Paper were abandoned in favour of local authority and voluntary hospitals remaining as executive units, surmounted by a regional and area system of planning. The regional councils (about ten in number) would, as expert advisory bodies, be based on university medical schools whilst the area planning authorities would roughly coincide with the envisaged joint authorities of the White Paper. The regional councils would be mainly concerned with hospital and specialist services but could criticize and advise on other health services, a remnant of the idea of a unified administrative system. The Area Planning Councils would prepare plans for all health services in their area. In addition in each area, there would be a hospital planning group, equally representative of voluntary and local authority hospitals together with some doctors, who would plan the hospital and specialist services in collaboration with the regional authorities. These plans would be submitted to the Area

67

Planning Councils for incorporation in their general plans which would then go to the Minister and the regional body for approval. An appeal machinery was also suggested. Although the detail is by no means complete we can see here the Minister's attempt to meet the demands for regionalism, for local authority ownership and for voluntary hospitals' equal share in the planning process. However complicated it appears, it must be conceded to be a masterpiece in the art of compromise. Bevan cut at its weakest point—ownership; but he took over some of the rest of this plan which had been constructed so painfully in the face of conflicting views.

As far as is known the County Councils Association accepted the plan and certainly the Association of Municipal Corporations preferred it to Bevan's proposals. For both of them regional authorities with no executive power were preferable to earlier alternatives. In this they clashed with the British Medical Association who wanted the regional authorities to draw up the original draft plans and to have certain powers of supervision. On this latter point however the local authority associations were adamant: they wanted local government control and initiative.

Except for a report from the Trades Union Congress General Council which wanted more local authority representatives on the hospital planning groups on the grounds that they had more beds, no other comments could be discovered. It is fair, therefore, to say that except for the continuing tussle between the medical profession and local government, a large measure of agreement with the main bodies had been reached. Willink had sought, with considerable success, to provide simultaneously a unified health service (in planning terms) to meet medical views, special advisory machinery to suit voluntary hospitals and executive power for both voluntary hospitals and local authorities.

(d) The National Health Service Bill

The War ended, the general election brought a new Government and a new Minister and eventually the National Health Service Bill. This proposed the transfer of all hospitals and their endowments to the Minister (except for the endowments of the teaching hospitals). The hospitals were to be administered by *ad hoc* bodies in a two-tier system: the planning guidance and control to be in the hands of Regional Hospital Boards, serving areas based on medical schools and the day to day administration to be carried out by Hospital Management Committees. Only in the case of the teaching hospitals was a special administrative machinery created, Boards of Governors who are not responsible, like Hospital Management Committees, to the Regional Hospital Boards.

During its passage through Parliament several amendments of minor importance were accepted. The annual income of the Hospital Endowments Fund (made up of the endowments of the nationalized hospitals) was intended to be shared among Boards, but was amended to include Hospital Management Committees as well, and the committees were given the right to keep endowments made subsequent to the passing of the Act. The powers of the Hospital Management Committees were strengthened against the Boards by a series of amendments in the House of Lords. In the main, the accepted amendments aimed to achieve a greater measure of decentralization and, as a result, greater powers and duties for the Hospital Management Committees.

The British Medical Association's response was twofold: to express dissatisfaction with the transfer of ownership and secondly to insist on safeguards against local government control creeping into the Regional Hospital Boards and Hospital Management Committees. One suspects however that their relief at getting the hospital service away from local government tended to outweigh their disappointment at the loss of voluntary hospitals. Most of the consultant members of the Association probably had a greater degree of welcome than sorrow for the Bill, as vouchsafed by the guarded welcome expressed for the Bill by the Royal College of Physicians. There is some strong evidence to suggest that the Minister deliberately set out to woo the consultants, perhaps thereby to break the medical opposition. He accorded the teaching hospitals a favourable position administratively and on their endowments, he instituted no disciplinary machinery for consultants (although he did so for general practitioners), he permitted the treatment of private patients for fees in state hospitals (despite backbench criticism from his own Party) and in some of the amendments he accepted in the Commons, he was falling in with the wishes of the Royal College. All in all he seems to have made a considerable attempt to win their support. As a result the general practitioners were, in a sense, deserted by their consultant colleagues and their position weakened.

As might be expected the County Councils Association could not welcome a Bill which took away their hospitals. They felt it not to be in accord with democratic principles to allow appointment to the administrative bodies rather than election. Local interest in the hospitals would diminish, and they felt it would be best to return to the 'position reached in consequence of the protracted negotiations'— i.e. the Willink Plan. The Association of Municipal Corporation followed, a day or two later, with very similar comments. The London County Council, with a Labour majority, was alone among the local authorities to welcome the Bill, but not without considerable heartsearchings. London was a special case to which we shall return in a later chapter.

The Local Government Associations with their long experience of contact with Government and Parliament, did not rest content with merely stating a case. Instead they prepared and, through their members in Parliament, sought to achieve a series of detailed amendments aimed not only at the selfish interest of local government, but also at improving the detail of the Bill. At no time did they descend to obstruction, and instead, whilst putting their point of view, sought to put their vast administrative experience at the call of Government to make technical improvements in the Bill.

The day before the Bill was published the British Hospitals Association produced a plan which represented a compromise between the Willink Plan and what they had presumably heard from the Minister of the contents of his Bill. They proposed considerably strengthening the powers of the regional authorities, to include the power to say what a hospital should do, but of course, with the current owners retaining their ownership. When the Bill had become public knowledge, the British Hospitals Association went on record as welcoming its aim, but as calling for the 'retention by the voluntary hospitals of their property and management, their entities and their tradition' as the only way to achieve an efficient service. When Bevan proved adamant, they were only left with a very minor role, joining in the call for more executive power at the periphery of the structure and changing the Bill with regard to the rights of committees to accept endowments after the Act had become law. As a group, once their property had gone, so had their bargaining powers.

In Parliament itself, Bevan had some minor differences with his own backbenchers over the 'concession' of pay beds in state hospitals, but no serious revolt developed. The Opposition, taking up the cudgels on the part of the Hospital Management Committees had some limited successes, but they were of a marginal kind, and they could hope for no major changes when faced by a minister with a huge Parliamentary majority at his back.

To review this chapter, we may note two conclusions. In the first place, Bevan's major contribution was the removal of ownership rights and with this, new solutions for the need for regional and local units, for co-ordination and development and for the removal of mutual local authority and voluntary hospital jealousies, became possible. His nationalization can be seen as a politically dogmatic action, or it can be seen as an inevitable result of the long negotiations and the unwieldy administrative structure proposed at the end of them. One cannot escape the conclusion that his decision probably owed more to the evident difficulties of the previous attempts than to his political views, although it is perhaps too much to have expected a Conservative minister to chose this solution.

The other major conclusion that stands here, as in other chapters, is due to the process of gradually filling in the details from plan to plan. The various attempts at unified control of all health services and at local control with some wider area provision which had changed to regionalism, together eventually brought a change of ownership, *ad hoc* regionalism and the complete separation of the hospitals from the other services. The discussion had come a long and unpredictable way from the original aims, shared by the Labour Party, of regional local government responsible for all health services.

6

General practitioner medical services

Writing this chapter at a time (1965) when the scene of the general practitioner service is in turmoil, when doctors are resigning or threatening to resign in large numbers, and when the word 'crisis' hangs heavily over all that is going on, it requires no stretch of the imagination to describe the general practitioner services as one of the most contentious elements in the discussion on the National Health Service. Contentious they were and are once again, a measure not only of the difficulties of 'employing' independent professional people, but also a comment on the fundamental insecurity of the general practitioner. What is a general practitioner and what is his job, why does he remain a *general* practitioner whilst all around him specialists both within and outside the medical profession multiply? Even when current disputes on the employment and remuneration of the general practitioner are solved, his future in a highly specialized medical service will remain a question.

To turn, however, to 1943. One great difference between the possible solutions for hospital and general practitioner services, was that although no acceptable administration for hospitals could be found without creating something new, in the general practitioner service there was an administrative structure for the National Health Insurance 'panel' system which represented the embodiment of another compromise between conflicting views (Braithwaite 1959). This system of Local Insurance Committees was the solution agreed after disputes between local government and the medical profession and as such was once again a potential resting place in the renewed conflicts between these two adversaries. As it was to turn out, this old compromise was to be the new compromise.

A series of problems faced the Government once they had decided on 100% coverage with the right of the patient to choose private practice if he so desired. The first was whether or not to allow the patient to choose his doctor, a right alleged by many people to be essential to the maintenance of the intimate trust of the doctor-patient relationship. As far as can be discovered, at no time did the Government envisage any modification or abrogation of this right, although on occasions, the British Medical Association had grave doubts of the Government's intentions. Under the National Health Insurance scheme, the general practitioner had been given the right to practise where he liked and to join if and when he so desired. This, however, did little to ensure a proper geographical distribution of doctors in relation to population, and the failure to achieve this was accepted as one of the weaknesses of the old system which the new scheme had to conquer. Two main alternatives presented themselves, either some form of compulsion or some form of attraction. It was possible to plan a scheme which directed doctors to where they should practise, or at least to refuse them the right to practise in areas already well provided with doctors, or it was possible to plan a scheme in which economic incentives were offered to attract doctors to under-doctored areas.

74

To do the latter involved the thorny issue of remuneration of general practitioners, an issue which today in 1965 has gone beyond the amount of remuneration once again to the method of remuneration. Under the National Health Insurance system the doctor was paid a gross annual fee (out of which he had to pay his own expenses) for each patient on his list and in return the doctor undertook to provide all proper and necessary general practitioner services. In 1943 there were those who supported this system as an incentive to good doctoring, whilst at the same time leaving the doctor free to organize his work to suit his professional needs without state interference or inspection. It was opposed by those who claimed that a doctor could only increase his income by overloading his list of patients and that he could only improve his lot by keeping expenses low to the detriment of the care he provided. For many of these opponents, the solution was a full-time salaried service which, for them, had the added advantages of cutting out what was in their view the anomalous position of the same doctors providing both public and private treatment —the dual standards of treatment, so called. The salary proposal was, however, anathema to many, if not most doctors on the grounds that it would make the doctor a civil servant, rob him of his professional independence and take away the safeguard of a separate private income. There were, of course, many other possible alternative methods of remuneration, but except for the two already mentioned and combinations of them, none of the other alternatives were seriously explored.

Another issue related to remuneration was that of the sale of the goodwill of National Health Insurance practices: prior to the Act of 1946 a new doctor entering a practice bought the goodwill of the practice built up by his predecessor. There were those who regarded this as wrong and the phrase 'the sale of patients in the medical market place' was often heard. But there were stronger objections to this system related, in part, to the desire for a salaried service but more strongly to the need to achieve a better geographical distribution of doctors. If some measure of direction or attraction were to be used, was it feasible to continue the sale of goodwill?

Traditionally the organization of general practice itself had been for a doctor to work on his own making his own arrangements for holidays, leisure time and so on. This led, said many critics, to the overwork and isolation of the general practitioner who had little time to keep up to date with medical advances by attending refresher courses or reading. There seemed a general measure of agreement that the solution to some of these problems lay in doctors' grouping together and sharing the work load to their and their patients' advantage. There were many who foresaw this grouping taking place in health centres, buildings in which all health services, except the institutional, would work together. If however this was to be so, the provision and running of these health centres was to be a matter of contention. Government proposals to make this a local government responsibility was seen by the medical profession as a back door method for setting up the hated local government control of general practitioners.

This raised, of course, the wider issue of the administration of these services and we have already noted the earlier compromise of 1911. The problems can best be stated in a series of questions. Was the administration to be national, regional or local? If all health services were under one unified administration then the problem of who should run the general practitioner services was solved: experience in the discussions was to prove the falsity of this hope, for what suited hospital administration and the groups concerned there did not suit general practitioner service administration and the groups concerned there. As time went on unification was ruled out, and so the question was whether to link general practitioner services to local government, to the hospital service or to a separate *ad hoc* administration. To try for unification in the administrative structure as several plans since 1948 have suggested, one must still provide satisfactory answers to these questions.

(a) The Brown Plan

Any minister, therefore, preparing this part of the National Health Service was moving into a territory beset on all sides with pitfalls. Emotions were strong and precipitate action could bring explosive results from at least some of the groups: this Brown found to his cost in 1943. He proposed a free general practitioner service available to all whilst preserving the right of the patient to choose his own doctor. The doctors, in urban areas at least, would work from health centres and be paid a full-time salary: new doctors would have to choose between full-time service or staying out of the scheme, whilst doctors already in practice would be allowed to retain the right to engage in part-time private practice. The services would be controlled by the local health authority who, together with a Central Medical Board, would make appointments to the general practitioner service. Here in simple terms was the full-time salaried local government service: it included almost everything that the British Medical Association hated most, and as a result they reacted violently against it. So speedy and strong was this reaction that few other groups had time to comment before the Minister had agreed to put his plan 'in the discard' and try again. One group, whose existence was threatened by the proposal, the National Association of Insurance Committees, joined the medical profession in condemning it. But for these bodies, few others commented on this plan.

77

(b) The White Paper

When Brown gave way to Willink, fresh thinking took place and the next version of the Government's plans appeared as the White Paper of 1944. This set down the principles which the Government felt should guide the planning of the service (all of which the medical profession accepted but claimed were invalidated by the actual proposals of the White Paper): the freedom of the doctor and the patient to use the service or not, with the contingent right of the patient to seek private treatment if he so desired, the right of the patient to choose his doctor, the freedom of the doctor to pursue his own professional methods without outside clinical interference and the preservation of the peculiar intimacy of the doctor-patient relationship.

The White Paper proposed the establishment of a central executive body (composed mainly of doctors) to be known as the Central Medical Board. The doctor entering the service would be under contract with this body and with the local authority if working in a health centre. The local duties of the Board would be exercised by local committees (including representatives of the local authority) and would supercede the Insurance Committees of the 'panel' system.

The general practitioner service would be freely available to all and although administrative responsibility would rest with the Central Medical Board, the joint authorities would be expected to make reference to these services in their area plans. The doctor would practise, singly, or in groups, or in health centres and would normally be remunerated on a capitation basis as before, but for those in health centres, remuneration would be by way of salary or other similar alternatives to avoid undesirable competition among centre doctors for patients. The doctor would be entitled to do part-time private work but newly

78

qualified doctors, if wanting to go into the public services, might, in certain areas, be required by the Board to work full-time in the public service for a number of years. Doctors newly entering or changing practice would have to seek the prior approval of the Central Medical Board with a view to achieving a better geographical distribution of doctors. Health centres would be provided and maintained by local authorities and the right to sell practices was left open for subsequent discussion.

Thus the White Paper rejected a full-time salaried local government service, although the local authorities were still in the picture with health centres, and through joint authorities, with the area plans. This was all that remained of the unified administration, at least from the point of view of the general practitioner services.

At first the medical profession's joint committee sought clarification on a number of issues, and key among them, was the power the Minister proposed for the Central Medical Board. The Minister reiterated the need for using the Board to affect a redistribution of doctors and insisted that the proposal for directed full-time service applied only to young doctors in certain areas—they could still go elsewhere or go into private practice. Further issues on which the profession posed questions concerned the control of health centres, the doctors suggesting joint authority rather than local authority control, whether or not they were to be regarded as experimental and the method of remuneration therein.

Subsequently in a more detailed critique of the White Paper, the British Medical Association rejected the powers of direction of the Central Medical Board, described the local organization as 'chaotic' and all in all saw the plans as the thin end of the wedge of a state salaried service. In return, they suggested that remuneration be the same in or out of health centres, that they first be established on

79

an experimental basis in a few areas, and that the compensation for the loss of practice value for those going into health centres (proposed by the White Paper) should be compensation for all doctors or none. At this stage, however, the tone was mild and statesmanlike although the gap between them and the Government was still very wide.

Other parts of the medical profession did not, however, share some of these views of the British Medical Association. The Socialist Medical Association deplored the British Medical Association's attitude and the Medical Practitioners Union described the report of the larger body as 'hesitating and obscure', 'nebulous and incomplete'. The Union felt that the Central Medical Board should be elected, that it should provide health centres and that doctors be allowed to choose between a full-time salaried service and a part-time capitation service. Remuneration should include allowances for length of service and special qualifications. With views like these, it is perhaps not surprising that the rest of the profession were not prepared to have the Union on its joint committee. How far each of these conflicting viewpoints was really representative is arguable and beyond the terms of reference of this book. Suffice it to note that a questionnaire filled in by members of the profession at this time suggested a far less united profession than its leaders claimed. The frequent references in medical politics to the need for unity suggested both that unity was not really there and also, points to the importance of an appearance of unity in the ranks for a pressure group in conflict with the Government.

Few other views on this section of the plan were expressed: it is, however, interesting to note the Trades Union Congress accepting a large part of the proposals only rejecting the continuation of the part-public, part-private practices of many doctors. In their report they go on to make the point of not pressing for a salaried service as the paramount need was the co-operation of the doctors. It is a tangential but interesting point to see the 'realistic' line adopted by the Trades Union Congress and to note from evidence gathered from a variety of sources, that they had consultations with and actually advised the medical profession how far they could reasonably expect to be able to push a Government.

(c) The Willink Plan

With the medical profession, therefore, far from satisfied, the discussions continued until the revision was circulated—the Willink Plan. In this plan the role and very existence of the Central Medical Board was challenged. Its powers of compulsion were gone and its existence left to the medical profession. Instead it was proposed, as an alternative, to return to a revised form of the Local Insurance Committees. The whole tenor of the plan was, in fact, to use as far as possible the National Health Insurance machinery and system, replacing the Local Insurance Committees with local committees of nominated representatives of the various professions together with some others. Local professional committees would also be established. Health centres would only be provided by local authorities as controlled experiments of the Central Health Services Council and the doctors working in them would be paid in the same way as those outside. The proposal of a part-salary element in the remuneration was raised for consideration by the profession. This could be varied to attract doctors to needy areas, the phrases used to justify this proposal being almost identical to those used later by Bevan as he sought to justify a similar proposal. The wider issues of remuneration were to be left to a committee (Spens 1946). On the sale of medical practices, the Government said the issues could be left until the service was in operation. With this plan, therefore, the wheel had turned full circle: the administration of the general practitioner service would revert to *ad hoc* machinery separate from other health services, remuneration was shelved, the powers of compulsion and direction dropped and health centres demoted to 'experiments'. The medical profession had clearly gained a big 'victory'.

This plan was soon accepted in all but a few details by the British Medical Association, but they insisted on adding further conditions before complete acceptance. Remuneration levels must be known, private practice safe-guarded, more information on the disciplinary machinery provided and the mechanics of the control of the issue of National Insurance sickness certificates set down, before the plans could be formally accepted. It is hard to resist the feeling that here the leaders of the British Medical Association were looking for further obstacles, making each a hurdle before adding another.

If the British Medical Association was satisfied, the Medical Practitioners' Union and the Socialist Medical Association can only be described as 'alarmed'. They saw the Willink Plan as reactionary and called for a return to the White Paper. At this time, the forthcoming general election led the Labour Party to publish its views on the general practitioner services. The sale of medical practices would be discontinued but compensation would be paid. Doctors would be paid a salary and be prohibited from private practice, but, as is so often the case in Party mani-festos, the wording is vague and may have meant some-thing less than this. Little or nothing was said of the type of administration to be adopted. It would be unfair to construe this as the Labour Party's answer to the Willink Plan but it does show some of the main points of differ-ence and no doubt could be taken as the writing on the wall of the future for the medical profession.

(d) The National Health Service Bill

The Bill took something from the Labour Party's plan and from the previous Willink Plan. In a sense, Bevan turned the wheel back somewhat but at the same time took over much of the helpful details of earlier plans. In the Bill, local *ad hoc* bodies (Local Executive Councils) would be set up to provide this service (and others) over areas corresponding to those of county and county borough councils. General practitioners would work mainly from health centres provided by the local authorities. The sale of medical practices would cease and compensation be paid. New doctors or doctors changing area would have to apply to the Medical Practices Committee for permission. There would be a disciplinary machinery headed by a central tribunal.

Thus Bevan followed the Willink Plan in settling for *ad hoc* machinery, he revived the idea of negative direction but without the power to compel full-time service from young doctors, he permitted the continuance of part-public, part-private practices, decided to end the sale of medical practices, restored health centres to the forefront and set up disciplinary machinery. All but the last point came from earlier plans, but on one issue he was silent. He refused to write into his Bill anything about the remuneration of general practitioners, a decision which caused considerable anxiety among the medical profession. On this point, Bevan defeated an Opposition amendment in the Commons, saw an amendment written in by the Lords and subsequently removed by the Commons because it 'was inexpedient that the method of remunerating doctors . . . be laid down in the Statute' and yet in 1949 introduced an amending Act which, *inter alia*, made the point of the amendment, i.e. the banning of remuneration by salary. This brief catalogue hides a long story running beyond our closing date in 1946 and telling of mounting medical opposition and a final concession by the Minister as the price of getting the service started.

This part of the Bill had a stormy passage through Parliament but suffered only few amendments, none of any consequence. The Opposition looked back to the Willink Plan and some members of the Labour Party regretted some of Mr. Bevan's 'concessions', in the main to no successful purpose. The real amendment was only to come with the Act of 1949 and also, perhaps, the failure to develop the health centres as intended in the years after 1948.

How did the groups react to the Bill? The British Medical Association regretted the three part administration calling rather for regional integration. As might be expected the Association objected to the compulsory powers of the Medical Practices Committee and to the abolition of the sale of goodwill which together with Bevan's mention of a part-salary element in their remuneration brought, they felt, the hated salaries service near. But for these major criticisms however, there was little else of moment in the Association's comments on this part of the Bill.

The Medical Practitioners Union found the Bill disappointing, feeling the status of the general practitioner to be debased: he would be cut off from hospital work, subject to disciplinary machinery not applicable to consultants, and his chances of teamwork in a health centre greatly impaired. The Socialist Medical Association, on the other hand, welcomed the Bill but regretted the lack of a salaried service and proposed that doctors in health centres should be paid by salary whilst those working outside should be able to opt for a salary.

As far as the medical profession was concerned there were several more battles before the service began to operate, and the eighteen months after the date which marks the end of the period studied here, saw further intense

84

discussions and negotiations. Its role in the discussions after 1948 has been well documented (Eckstein 1960) but the period between 1946 and 1948 has received little attention as yet.

Little more remains in this chapter. In the local government world the two major associations disagreed on health centres, the Association of Municipal Corporations saying they should be Regional Hospital Board responsibilities because of the heavy cost and limited local authority powers, whilst the County Councils Association welcomed the proposals in the Bill but called for increased power for local authorities saying that doctors working in these centres should be local government officials. A welcome, with some qualifications, came from the National Association of Insurance Committees for the proposals which in effect served to bring them back from the limbo of earlier plans.

In conclusion we can note how far the discussion had moved away from a salaried local government service as part of the unified health administration. Gradually a separate administration crept in and all the old (and often allegedly unsuccessful) National Health Insurance elements came back. Bevan had his own Party to placate so he reversed the trend somewhat but he went only a small part of the way back to Brown. The most 'socialist' plan came from the Liberal National minister, whilst only a middle of the road plan came from the Labour minister: an odd political paradox as a memorial to the power of the medical pressure group. They had not won complete victory, but it could have been much worse—and there were further gains to be recorded later.

7

Other general practitioner services

The National Health Service Act groups together for administrative purposes, the general practitioner medical services, the general dental pharmaceutical and ophthalmic services. In the case of the pharmaceutical services, these had been an integral part of the National Health Insurance system whilst the other two were available to some contributors as additional benefits: i.e. those extra benefits available to the contributors of approved societies whose funds were sufficiently in surplus. There was, thus, in all three cases some experience of national provision, however limited the scale.

The problems facing the Minister with these three services only emerged gradually; at first they were treated as little more than appendages to the general practitioner medical service. Leaving aside the administrative issues which were very similar to those already discussed in the previous chapter, the main issues seemed to be professional. The dentists were concerned about achieving independence from the medical profession, were worried about the talk of employing ancillary workers in dental surgeries and were upset at the prospect of continuing control of

86

their more expensive work—under National Health Insurance schemes they had had to submit prior estimates of expensive work before starting on the treatment. The pharmacist, too, had professional problems: the over-supply of pharmacists, the need to engage in the sale of cosmetics and the like to achieve a living and the resultant public image of the shop counter chemist. The opticians were in dispute with the doctors: as lay people they claimed the right to test eyes and prescribe glasses (as well as actually making them) but the medical profession claimed that testing and prescribing was a medical function and not one for lay people untrained in the wider symptomology of bodily disease. All in all, they were a nervous trio, all anxious to use the opportunity of the creation of a National Health Service to establish full and secure professional status.

(a) The Brown Plan

The first Government plan seems not to have gone into the details which would include these services, so there is little direct comment from the groups to record. There is, however, plenty of evidence to suggest that the plan, if it did nothing else, stirred these three professions to examine their own positions. One obvious fact about dentistry was the shortage of dentists: a fact which was conceded by the Government with the appointment of the Teviot Inter-Departmental Committee (Teviot 1944) to review the stages by which a dental service could be introduced in the light of such a shortage, the steps necessary to increase the intake of dental students and the government and control of the dental profession. The appointment of this committee seemed to calm the fear of the British Dental Association that doctors would represent them in the discussion with the Ministry of Health. (At this time and indeed until 1956, the profession's controlling body, the General

87

Dental Council, was virtually only a committee of the General Medical Council). The British Dental Association, thus assured, set out its views in a memorandum to the Teviot Committee. These views can be summed up as follows: freedom from medical control, no salaried service of local or central government and the maintenance of private practice. The patients would be divided into two classes: priority classes (i.e. children and young persons up to the age of eighteen and nursing and expectant mothers) to be treated in dental health centres run by the Ministry of Health and the non-priority classes to be treated by general dental practitioners working from their own surgeries. Dentists in the former would be paid by salary and the latter either by a scale of fees for work done for patients over the age of eleven when the scheme began, or, subsequently when the service was established, for persons who had been through the priority service and were dentally fit at the age of eighteen, a *per capita* fee for each patient on the dentist's list. The underlying assumption here was that a young person who had been made dentally fit by the priority service, needed an easily calculable amount of treatment each year, hence making a *per capita* fee possible. The naivety of this assumption has subsequently been shown by studies of the incidence of dental disease even among young adults and by the considerable undermanning in the 'priority' services. The British Dental Association however saw its proposals as making possible a gradual advance to a full service.

Meantime the pharmacists were calling, as we have seen earlier, for a separate pharmaceutical organization to run their service and the opticians were recalling the long history of the disputes with the medical profession over sight testing. They also took the opportunity to call for full State registration of opticians, one of the legal hallmarks of a fully fledged profession.

(b) The White Paper

When the White Paper was published in 1944, little was added to the proposals for these services; in fact little was said of them at all. The British Dental Association took the opportunity to challenge earlier systems whereby expensive treatment had been subject to control, for the dentist should have the professional freedom to decide the appropriate treatment without control. (As an example, the case of gold fillings may be quoted. In terms of dental health 'ordinary' fillings might be sufficient, but the patient may prefer the aesthetic advantages of gold fillings. It was the freedom to provide these gold fillings which, *inter alia*, the profession was anxious to have.) The Association reiterated its call for a separate dental organization and declared that it was opposed to geographical direction of any kind.

By the end of 1944 the Teviot Committee had produced an Interim Report (Teviot 1944) calling for a comprehensive service based on a dental equivalent of the family doctor service, whilst the priority classes should be provided for by the local authorities. The Report, together with the White Paper, brought the dental profession fully into practical discussions on the future of their services.

The White Paper's proposals to continue the supply of drugs and medicines through chemists shops and primarily by qualified pharmacists was thankfully welcomed by the profession. They were less happy with the non-appearance of a pharmaceutical organization and of any proposals to control entrance to their profession. They set out in considerable detail proposals for a separate administration for their service and said they wanted security from unjust competition, proper remuneration (but not a salary) and freedom from 'undue' lay interference. The details in the Government's planning had not gone far enough for this group to get involved in deep discussion, so they were left making grandiose claims to all who would listen.

A similar comment applies to the opticians: they contented themselves by setting out four principles. The public should have the right to choose between public and private services, the practitioners should have freedom in their professional work, private practice should continue and finally the practitioner should have the choice of working in the service, in private practice or both. They, too joined the queues claiming a separate administrative structure.

(c) The Willink Plan

By the time the Willink Plan of 1945 was being circulated, the details had been painted in and they looked remarkably like a revised version of the National Health Insurance system. The administration of the three services (except for the priority dental services which would be a local authority responsibility) would be the duty of *ad hoc* local committees which would also run the general practitioner medical services. The 'economic' control of expensive dental treatments would rest with a central dental board. A Spens Committee (Spens 1948) would be set up to consider dental remuneration on the lines of the similar committee for general medical practitioners.

Much of this plan seemed to please the dental profession, particularly the offer of a Spens Committee. The dentists accepted the central board and called for more dental representatives on the Central Health Service Council. They did however, take the apparently selfish position of saying that agreement on remuneration must precede any formal acceptance of the administrative proposals. So, despite this general agreement, they preferred to wait on the remuneration proposals before finally agreeing.

The pharmacists, too, accepted the proposals but called for more seats on the local *ad hoc* committees. In subsequent discussions at the Ministry of Health they received assurances on the importance of pharmaceutical advice in the administrative structure at national and local levels, that pharmaceutical work should be done only by qualified pharmacists and that the position of the chemists' shops would be safeguarded.

For the opticians, no comment could be discovered and it is likely that the dispute between medical and lay opticians was still making a decision difficult. But, by reverting to the National Health Insurance system and modifying it to take account of the increased population to be covered, the increased number of professions concerned and the disappearance of the Approved Societies of the system Willink had secured a large measure of agreement on these services.

(d) The National Health Service Bill

The National Health Service Bill followed in large measure the Willink plan. Local Executive Councils which would include representatives of these professions would be responsible for the services, except for priority dental services which would be a local authority responsibility. A Dental Estimates Board would be set up to consider dentists' estimates for the more expensive types of treatment. In the case of the ophthalmic services, the Minister considered that sight-testing and prescribing eventually should be Regional Hospital Board responsibilities, but until enough ophthalmic surgeons were available, it would be necessary to create temporary committees, linked with executive councils, to provide what was called the Supplementary Ophthalmic Services. Little amendment of any consequence was made to the Bill in this context during its passage through Parliament.

The dental reactions to the Bill were of vociferous opposition to it. The Dental Estimates Board displeased greatly, as surprisingly did the proposal that priority dental services be the duty of local authorities (the Association had earlier proposed this themselves). They objected to the implications of dentistry's being forced into health centres. They found the Minister high-handed in his dealings with them, but after the Bill became law, they confessed themselves somewhat mollified by later discussions with the Minister. Their basic sense of insecurity however remained, for as they said in one of their handout leaflets, 'if all the amendments had been obtained, however generous the remuneration and however acceptable the conditions of service may appear, the position of the profession will still be insecure . . .' As an example of the sensitivity to insecurity, an editorial in the British Dental Journal referred to 'the most disquieting feature' of the Parliamentary discussions —the 'irresponsible and uninformed suggestions put forward by Mr. Willink as to the possible dilution of the profession by persons who have received no recognized training'. In a sentence, the dentists no doubt felt it could have been much worse, but the writing they saw on the wall boded ill.

The pharmacists felt unhappy about health centres, *inter alia*, but most of their doubts were relatively minor ones. Like the other professions they unsuccessfully sought amendments to the Bill, but unlike dentists, on the whole, they felt their professional status was more secure as a result of the Bill and therefore had, in the main, favourable views on the plans.

As for the opticians, the temporary solution left them dissatisfied and with the strong feeling that the real and decisive battle was still to come. As this is written in 1965, nearly twenty years afterwards, the temporary solution begins to look more and more permanent and, at long last, the Ministry has, in the marked absence of any increase in the number of medically qualified ophthalmic surgeons, either now or in the near future, indicated its willingness

92

to make the temporary solution permanent. The battle is therefore more or less over and the lay opticians have won.

To sum up this chapter, we may say that most of the disputes were domestic to the groups concerned, for rarely did the larger groups, such as the medical profession, comment on the various proposals. The outline of the various plans shows that once the broader outlines of the National Health Service began to fall into shape along three separate organizations, so it was possible to fill in the details of these services. Important though each was (and still is) in its own way, they were only relatively minor details in the total picture. The logical progression from broad outline to detail, meant these services were late entrants into the proposals and indeed many of the disputes of the three services came into the open only after the passage of the Act made it possible to begin the detailed process of drawing up regulations. In this book, we stop short at the Royal Assent to the Act, but policy making (at a lower level) went on, in consultation with the groups, right up to the date of the inauguration of the service on July 5, 1948.

8

Local authority health services and the mental health services

Little purpose would be served by making this chapter a long one : many of the issues concerned here revolve around the type of administrative structure to be adopted and less around the services to be provided. In addition to ambulance and health centre duties, the National Health Service Act laid on county and county borough councils what might be described as the personal preventive services, including a limited role in the care and after care of domicilary illness. Most of these duties represent little more than extensions of existing functions, although the health centre and ambulance duties were new to local government.

The problem facing the Government here was twofold. If a unified administration was to be achieved, was it to be a local government system? If unification should prove impossible, was there a role for local authorities and if so what was it? Was it to include the continued provision of hospitals and institutional services, was it to include only public health duties, or something in between? The two major stumbling blocks the Government had to face were the unreformed and allegedly inefficient system of

94

local government and the hatred, hardly too strong a word, of the medical profession (and most of the other professions as well) of local government control of their services.

The chapter heading includes reference to the mental health services but these are reserved for a brief discussion at the end of the chapter. This is not to decry their importance, but rather to make the point that the growing demand that mental illness be more and more integrated with physical illness in its treatment services, meant that little especial consideration was given to this service. One point, however, does emerge on this service of some generic importance. Up to 1946 the local authorities had been responsible for both the domicilary and institutional care of the mentally ill. To split the administrative structure of the National Health Service as a whole between institutional and other types of care, meant breaking this allegedly ideal unity under local government.

(A) Local Health Authority services

(a) The Brown Plan

To take up the development of local authority services with the Brown Plan, the solution proposed was a deceptively simple one : Joint Health Boards of combined local authorities were to be responsible for all health services. The Boards were to be a temporary expedient pending the reform of local government. As we have seen the medical profession's reaction to this idea was immediate and completely negative. For the local government side, the County Councils Association could not agree to its loss of executive responsibility to these Joint Boards, and instead called for a greater measure of constituent local authority control over them. The County Councils wanted as far as possible to keep the local authorities in control, especially for the services they were already running: they resented, as they almost always do, the loss of powers.

(b) The White Paper

The next plan, the White Paper, proposed joint authorities which would, it was suggested, set out the relationship between themselves and the constituent authorities in their area plans, but as a general rule it was laid down that what we now know as local health authority services would be the executive responsibility of the local authorities, except in the cases of the ambulances which would be a joint authority responsibility. These authorities would be composed of local government representatives with an advisory machinery on the lines of local versions of the proposed Central Health Services Council. This relatively minor role for the professions as advisers was, as has been noted, rejected by the medical and some of the other professions. Local government, on the other hand welcomed the exclusion of the professions on the ground that to have included them would have been a dangerous impairment of the principle of public responsibility. Both the County Councils Association and the Association of Municipal Corporations felt that the joint authorities should be limited only to planning and have no executive functions. They saw the proposals as the thin end of the wedge of regionalism in local government which they were determined to prevent, if at all possible. Later the County Councils Association went further, saying that local health services should in no way at all be a responsibility of the joint authority. As the major associations were fighting to keep their services, the associations of the smaller local authorities were making another point. The Urban District Councils Association which protested against joint authorities *and* against any concentration of executive health powers in the hands of county councils. Enterprising and progressive

96

urban districts should be given or retain certain health powers, particularly those in the maternity and child welfare field. Thus local government had no unified voice and without it, it had less chance to convince the ministers of the virtue of local government as an executive element in the National Health Service.

It is worth noting the special case of London at this point. Willink proposed to concentrate all local authority health services in the London area under the London County Council to the exclusion of the Metropolitan Boroughs, the second tier of London government. This, quite naturally, the boroughs objected to as 'the foundation stones of local government in London'. Subsequent discussions with the Minister came to an end with a compromise to the effect that, although the powers be given to the London County Council, it would be compelled to delegate them to the boroughs. To jump ahead of our chronology, the Metropolitan Boroughs' Standing Joint Committee and the London County Council agreed, after Bevan's arrival, to submit this plan to him for inclusion in his Bill. Leading the Metropolitan Boroughs' deputation was their Chairman, Alderman C. Key, who later, as the Parliamentary Secretary to the Minister of Health, found himself in the unique and difficult position of refusing to accept the plan he had earlier canvassed—a situation fully savoured and enjoyed by the Opposition in Parliament.

(c) The Willink Plan

To revert to the White Paper, it had sought to make hospitals and ambulances a joint authority responsibility and the other local health services a local authority responsibility. A year or more later, in the Willink Plan, the *supra*-local authority machinery was reduced to planning with no executive functions and all the executive functions were to remain with county and county borough councils. Each authority would be required to co-opt doctors to a statutory health committee. Most of this plan, naturally enough, pleased the major local authority associations who, by now, had moved on to concentrate on administrative details, the grant system, the responsibility of local authorities for non-residents and so on—the bread and butter of local government work in any service. Up to this point, the major local authorities had done well, they had lost no powers and had gained more. Regionalism was gone, the joint authority system was almost powerless and the professions kept out of executive control. Everything in the local government garden seemed rosy.

(d) The National Health Service Bill

The next plan, whilst making local authorities responsible for all local health authority services as well as ambulances, took away their powers over hospitals. In this they lost an important service. The County and County Borough Councils had to appoint health committees and co-opt doctors onto these committees. The Association of Municipal Corporations successfully joined the Associations of smaller authorities, in claiming that county councils should be compelled or allowed to delegate some of their duties to second tier authorities. In the London area too, the Minister had to resist attempts to write delegation into his Bill. We cannot say with certainty why this was so, particularly as Alderman Key was one of the health ministers, but a reasonable guess runs along these lines: Bevan probably began, like Willink, by thinking of London as a single hospital region with the London County Council as the authority, or at least playing a large part. This, however, would have been strongly resisted by the medical profession and the voluntary hospitals who in earlier discussions had talked of splitting up London into several regions

98

stretching out into the Home Counties to widen the influence of teaching hospitals. Whether it was the logic of this or the need to please the consultant section of the profession is not clear, but Bevan's decision to make four regions in London meant that the London County Council could no longer play any major or influential part in the Regional Hospital Board structure. It could be, therefore, that the refusal to accept delegation, together with the additional (and illogical) duty of providing an ambulance service, were part of the sop to a disappointed London County Council and to its great personality and fellow Cabinet Minister, Herbert Morrison. In his endeavours to meet the medical profession Bevan had, both in London and elsewhere, to disappoint local government but he tried to soften the blow (to some extent).

As might be expected the local authority associations were not happy with many of the proposals of the Bill, but it is interesting to note that, although they tried for some major amendments of principle, they also (unlike many other groups) concentrated on suggesting many detailed amendments which their experience as administrators of past Acts of Parliament suggested as necessary. Although they often took up what can only be described as sectional positions, they also performed the vital service of applying their wealth of experience and administrative skill to a detailed study of the Bill. As such, whatever one may think of their sectional interests, they were performing a useful and necessary democratic function in policy making.

In the end the local government system came out the loser, but the development of plans over the four years shows that attempts were made to move nearer to its viewpoint and the end result was, in some considerable measure, due to its pressures, discussions and existence. But for the local governments the structure of the National

Health Service might have been very different and if, in the future, it is to be different again, it will have to be both with them and in spite of them.

(B) The Mental Health Services

To conclude this chapter with a brief glance at the mental health services, we must be dogmatic and dangerously uncomplicated in a territory where the State has had a long history of legislative interference in one way or another (Jones 1955). In 1939 the bulk of provision for the care of the mentally ill and mentally handicapped rested with local government. Central responsibilities were divided between the Ministry of Health and the Board of Control. The legislation which governed these services and responsibilities was long and involved, so much so that the task of reviewing the legislation and services seemed to Ernest Brown to be a formidable one. He decided, therefore, not to include the mental health service in his plan for a National Health Service, a decision which the British Medical Association roundly condemned. Willink was braver and in his White Paper he restated the difficulties of reforming the laws governing the mental health services, but declared that the Government was determined to include them : 'The aim must be to reduce the distinction drawn between mental ill-health and physical ill-health and to accept the principle declared by the Royal Commission on Mental Disorder that the treatment of mental disorder should approximate as nearly to the treatment of physical ailments as is consistent with the special safeguards which are indispensable when the liberty of the subject is infringed' (White Paper 1944). The White Paper proposed that all mental health services, institutional and non-institutional, should be the responsibility of the joint authorities.

Of this proposal little was specifically said by the groups that has not already been mentioned in other wider contexts, beyond one or two voices raised for a full review of the law in this field. In the Willink Plan of 1945 the mental health services were transferred to local authority control and again no specific comment is available. Bevan's Bill followed the previous two plans by including mental health services and trying to approximate them and their administration to the physical health services. For the mental health services this meant splitting institutional and non-institutional services between *ad hoc* hospital bodies and the local authorities. Again few specific comments were made : indeed the general lack of comment throughout may be related to two facts : the widespread ignorance and lack of interest in these services and the declared principle to treat them in the same way as the other services meant that little attention was devoted specifically to the mental health services. It could also be that the virtual dominance of the local authorities in this field and the consequent absence of strong voluntary groups and contingent medical loyalties, took away the major spokesmen on other hospital and health proposals. Whatever the reason, the result is clear : if the mental health services were to be little different, then they had to suffer the same administrative divisions as the other health services. It was not until much later, after the creation of the service, that the mental health services came into the limelight with a much more detailed analysis and review which culminated in the Mental Health Act, 1959 (Jones 1960). The calls for review of the legislation, the modernization of the concepts of and services for the treatment and care of the mentally ill, were not met until the service was some eleven years old.

9
Conclusions

The foregoing chapters summarize the findings of a detailed study of one aspect of the development of the National Health Service. In so doing, we may have overstated the importance and power of the pressure groups and may have undervalued, thereby, other important factors such as public opinion, *ad hoc* groups and so on. What is asked of the reader is that he sees this study in the wider context of a full history of the National Health Service and in the context of social policy making. It is abundantly clear that, when all the other factors are taken into account, and principles and logic satisfied, there were still some groups who had to be placated or convinced, for without them the service would never have started. How, then, in this chapter can we conclude on the development of the plans and the groups that were involved? Two aims will be attempted: one is to seek some balance sheet of success and failure for the groups concerned and the other is the overall development of the plans for a service.

There is no doubt whatever that *The Lancet* was right when it said in 1946 that the Act derived 'more from the long discussion between the profession and the Ministry of Health than it does from any doctrinaire idea of the . . . Minister's party'. Pressure groups are part of social policy making although perhaps even now in this case study, we cannot be certain as to how big a part they played. We can see how the plans changed, and where the changes are in the direction of the views of a pressure group, it is fair to claim some part for that group. Even where the changes are not obvious one can read of ministerial 'intentions' at a later stage which concede a pressure group's viewpoint. To do all this, however, the minister must have some ideas of his own (or from his officials), from which he could, if he so desired, have moved 'outwards' to meet the groups, a process once described rather cynically as a 'process of erosion'.

Brown was at the beginning of this process. His officials had a plan which aimed at regionalism, a tidy unified administrative structure, a salaried general practitioner service and a comprehensive range of services freely available to all. Much of this he had to put in the discard because of medical opposition, thereby depriving himself and his successor of a starting point, so Willink had to start again; as he said in a lecture late in 1944:

I sometimes feel that it must be depressing for those with whom we have had conversations . . . that in the first months when a project of this sort is under discussion, the Minister . . . has . . . nothing to give, no terms to make no promises. I think, however, that those who are experienced have understood that until a certain stage has been reached when we have an impression of the views of all concerned, we cannot begin to review the public mind as a whole, the views of the . . . (groups) and reshape to the right extent the original proposals.

In his White Paper of 1944 the process of erosion had begun. Many aims admittedly remained the same, but the

103

search for unified administration had become less sure, regionalism had been badly dented and the role of local government had diminished. At the same time we can see the development and the filling in of details. The proposal for a central medical board, for example, was a development made necessary by the abandonment of local government control of general practitioners. Local authorities would have had establishment figures and through them doctors would have been better distributed. At the same time, this second plan was able to go into more detail, some of the lesser services getting a mention.

By the Willink Plan of 1945 the central administrative and advisory machinery had been hammered out, but the idea of unification had almost gone. In its place, specialized administrations or planning units were creeping in and regionalism in the hospital world being developed. The remuneration of general practitioners was being explored as was the role of health centres. Development and detail went hand in hand. Then came Bevan who had to meet a new group, his own Party, and so went back on some of the changes resuscitating older ideas, taking over much of what had gone before and in the end adding only one new major feature the transfer of the ownership of hospitals. By now unification (except as a pious hope in health centres) had been abandoned and political realities overcame idealism to make a tripartite system using two existing systems and one new one. Aneurin Bevan was less of an innovator than often credited: he was at the end, albeit the important and conclusive end, of a series of earlier plans. He 'created' the National Health Service but his debts to what went before were enormous. In this case, as no doubt in others, great social policy decisions do not come down inscribed on sacred tablets from some political party's research centre, some government department or some idealist reformer: they are, rather, built up in discussion and negotiations—sometimes over short periods, sometimes, as in this case, over longer ones. Here it is quite clear that the original Government aims like those of the victorious Labour Party of 1945 had to be progressively modified or eroded to meet the conflicting views of the groups most concerned.

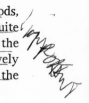

The groups' successes and failures

How did the various groups come out of the discussions? Without doubt the groups with skills to offer, particularly the medical profession, did best. Viewing the Act of 1946 against the plans of 1943, they had achieved a lot—no salaried service, no local government control, modified powers of direction, the removal of all hospitals from local government, and for the consultant, regionalism, special treatment for teaching hospitals, seats on the administrative bodies, no disciplinary machinery. Although general practitioners lost the right to sell their practices, and got a form of negative direction and a disciplinary system, all were better than the original 1943 plans. Indeed subsequent development since 1946 suggests that, except on remuneration, the medical profession has, by and large, prospered in its dealings with the Ministry of Health. 'We have the doctors: you want the doctors', one British Medical Association Chairman publicly told the Minister at an annual meeting of the Association. 'Crude pressure group stuff' or 'political realities', the Minister could not ignore it and sought to gain peace by compromise. The other professions, with the possible exception of the dentists, were less spectacularly successful, but still successful on a shorter list of credit balances. The Government had to assume the groups spoke for their members or run the calculated risks of dissension within the groups.

Weakest in this sense was the medical profession which

always felt that the 'defeat' on the National Health Insurance Act of 1911 was due to disunity in its own ranks. Even today (1965) as it flexes its muscles against yet another Minister, the same doubts are there; will all the doctors resign when asked, or when the crunch comes, will many concede the power of the almost monopolistic employer and stay on? Although they had the crucial skills the State needed in 1948, the medical profession's own divisions made it less strong than it might have been. Bevan saw its weaknesses and by wooing the consultants split the medical opposition in a very effective way.

Groups whose bargaining weapon was an administrative structure and skill were in a less powerful position. Where, as in the case of Insurance Committees, they represented an earlier compromise, they were at risk if the balance of power had changed, but when, as it eventually turned out, things were much the same as they had been in 1911, they could, in effect, offer their compromise for a second time. They did and survived. Where, like local government, they represented a structure always available for services seen to need local administration (perhaps with the added virtues of local democratic control), their position was somewhat different. Local government would not disappear or change just because of the National Health Service: local authorities would still be there with or without health services. They had, therefore, to stress the advantages of their system, of local democratic control and the virtues of all that they had previously done in the health field. Although the major authorities kept most of their services, except of course hospitals, and gained others, the smaller authorities lost such health services as they had had. When viewed against the Brown Plan of 1943 when local government would have been supreme (even if some of the existing authorities had disappeared) the final result, for the local government system was far from satisfactory. Counties and county boroughs were mollified, to some extent, but local government as a whole lost its potentially dominating role in the health services.

The groups with property to offer, the hospital groups, were in a powerful position whilst their rights of ownership were respected (although the financial arrangements could have undermined that position). Once, however, the decision was taken to nationalize their property, they ceased to count and in this context lost all. Against Conservative ministers without thoughts of nationalization, they were reasonably safe, but against a nationalizing Government they were almost inevitably doomed, especially when the earlier plans had demonstrated the administrative contortions that were necessary to meet their viewpoints.

This, then, is the brief balance sheet of success and failure as far as the groups were concerned at the time when the Royal Assent was given to the Act in November, 1946. Their gains and losses since that date could well be the subject of another study. At this point, however, the reader may care to ask himself how far he would view these 'successes' and 'failures', this 'process of erosion' from the vantage point of the 1960s and nearly twenty years of the service. Were the compromises the right or best ones, were too many 'concessions' made—or not enough? Studies of the development of the service since 1948 might well, at some date, provide some of the answers.

Pressures today

Many books have been written (although surprisingly few by British authors) on the development of the service since 1948 and many more no doubt remain to be written. This chapter is not an attempt to correct or evaluate those who have so far put pen to paper, nor is it an attempt to fill in the gaps in our knowledge of this development. Instead we wish to spotlight some of the trends and pressures revealed in this study and glance at their relevance today. The aim is suggestive, selective and speculative and in no sense definitive or comprehensive.

We have been concerned so far with the groups arrayed before the Government in the 1940s but it is rewarding to move beyond 1946 and see the changes which have taken place among the groups since then. In doing so two conclusions can be drawn : one is that most of the groups of 1946 are still flourishing and, although their views have mellowed and changed somewhat on the National Health Service, many of their more basic views (including those that caused all the difficulties in the war-time discussions) still remain. The medical profession on the whole remains opposed to local government, to 'interference in clinical matters', to a salaried service and to direction. These views may have a new clothing as befits the situation of the 1960s, but at heart they remain the same. Local government, too, remains opposed to regionalism and *ad hoc* bodies, favours keeping what it has and would like more; and so we could go on.

The other conclusion to be drawn from a survey of the groups today is the growth of new groups. In this two main trends can be instanced. In the first place there has been a growth of new organizations within the major groups. To take medicine as an example, there has been evidence of dissatisfaction with the part played by the major group, the British Medical Association, shown in the establishment of groups like the General Practitioners Association. There has been, too, a concern to improve the status of the general practitioner as seen in the setting up of the College of General Practitioners on the lines of the Royal Colleges for the consultant sections. The medical scene is changing and the weight and importance of the

108

new and older groups has yet to be established. The second trend in the establishment of new groups has been the creation of groups to safeguard the new administrative structures. In the executive council world, there is now the Executive Councils Association together with, *inter alia*, a body representing their Clerks. In the hospital world there is now an Association of Hospital Management Committees together with many groups representing their specialist officers. The groups in the administrative areas have thus proliferated to a considerable extent.

These new administrative groups, of course, are related to the once new structures. The structures are by now, however, no longer new: they are becoming more and more firmly embedded in the history of the health service and are steadily building up loyalties and support resistant to any change. To visit, as the author has done, conferences of the separate sections, is to find agreement on the need to get away from the tripartite structure and back to some kind of unification. But there the agreement ends: like local government in the 1940s all are in favour of change as long as they are the beneficiaries. To make a change now will disappoint some groups and any Minister seeking changes will have to count the corns on which he will have to tread. There is, too, the further point that there are those who now believe that a health service is too big an organization for one body and that sectionalization is inevitable, even if the current version is not the acceptable one. If, however, the efficient running of the service is to take precedence over the conflicting interests, little can be done without experiment and more knowledge. To make national changes without this may be only to make things worse. Perhaps the time has come to try some area experiments; e.g. let the hospital authorities in Area A run the ambulance service, let the executive council in area B provide health centres and in Area C try something else, and in each case measure the results. Change in a structure which is ossifying in its mould like the National Health Service will only come if there is a need for change and when knowledge and a forceful minister come together. Neither has so far happened.

Key figures in the National Health Service are obviously the professions who provide the care, but this, among social services, is by no means unique. What is unique in the service is the extent to which the professional workers have secured seats on the controlling bodies. Up to one quarter of hospital bodies, nearly a half of executive councils are professionals working for the committees they sit on. For example, a comparison with education shows the 'workers' there forbidden seats on their controlling committees. Is the difference a comment on the role that the layman can play in the National Health Service or on the strength of the professional groups? The plethora of committees in the service takes up the time of many laymen (as well as professionals) and poses the question both of the number of committees and the role of the laymen therein. Is the National Health Service an example of the trend in social policy of the growing technicalities of social provision which gives diminishing scope for a useful lay contribution?

The lay figure is on the committees to fulfill two potential roles. He is presumably the spokesman of the patient, the representative of the consumer (it is interesting to see the recent development of some small 'patient' groups such as the Association for the Improvement of Maternity Services or the Patients Association). To be a doctor and represent medical views is to represent a continuing group, but to be fit and represent the transient patient is much more difficult. (It would be instructive to discover how many members of these committees have been patients of the services they control.) The lay person may also be there in another role : to bring the lay contribution, whatever that may be, to the administration. He may be chosen because of the experience or expertise he can bring, but, by the methods of selection, this may often turn out to be his ability to 'represent' other groups or services. Does the layman make a contribution which is valuable in itself, or valuable as a spokesman for other group interests (including the patient) or is he there simply as a preventive to complete professional control?

Many changes have come onto the professional scene since 1948 and only a few can be touched on. A key one, which is far too large a topic to explore here, is the changing pattern of medical care. Wherever one looks there are examples of this. There is the increasing use of hospitalization and the growing importance of the consultant. There are the counter trends emphasizing domicilary care—earlier discharge from hospital, home confinements, community care in the mental health service are examples—either as the expression of ideals or, as is often suspected, the economic answer to the cost and shortage of hospital facilities. There is the peculiar position of general practice, the 'cottage industry of medicine' fighting to keep its status and role. Group practice had developed widely but health centres have not. General practitioners have lost many of their beds in hospitals, but are told they are the leaders of the domicilary team, many of whom are employed by other agencies. General practice is, or should be, undergoing an 'agonizing reappraisal'.

A key problem in all these issues which the National Health Service has had to face is the problem of the employment of professionals. To be a professional man implies being able, *inter alia*, to decide the treatment best suited to the patient. To do this, in the National Health Service, involves the spending of public monies and as the cost of the service rises, the question of controlling the activities of these people becomes more and more acute. One clash of interests involves the cost of prescribing and the general practitioner's right to prescribe as he thinks fit. It is at this point that increasing concern over the cost comes most painfully on a sensitive nerve of the professional groups. There is potential here for many more professional group conflicts with the Government.

There is, too, the phenomenon of the growth of new professions: the Professions Supplementary to Medicine Act 1961 gave Parliamentary blessing to six such. There are also signs of other new professions sprouting their wings, such as the hospital administrators whose qualifications and length of training is now beginning to rival that of the doctor. All these groups (and many more) mark out the new pressure points in the National Health Service and incidentally pose increasing problems for the hitherto unified and undisputed master profession of medicine. To the sociologist the National Health Service of recent years, and increasingly in the future, will prove a fruitful field for the study of the growth and proliferation of professions.

Finally in this projection of 1946 into the 1960s we can note the position of local government still virtually unchanged since 1946. Attempts at reform have largely been stillborn, although the recent activities of the Local Government Commission suggests some changes and the Local Government Act of 1958 has brought some increases in the powers of delegation of duties to second tier authorities in country areas. Basically, however, local government has the same strengths and weaknesses as in 1946, which give it both the grounds for calling for a continuing role, but at the same time an inability to tackle anything greater in the health field.

The pressures of the 1940s which have been discussed, remain, modified but probably basically the same. To amend the Act now might be to risk re-fighting old battles or it might demonstrate how almost twenty years of the service have modified the views of 1946. Change is not and ought not to be impossible if the service is to meet new problems. But the 'realities' that faced Bevan and his ministerial predecessors and were part of the decision-making process of 1946, serve as a warning even today for those who follow solely the 'dictates of abstract principles'.

Bibliographical notes

A study such as this one is the product of the compilation of data from many sources. Some of these sources, to which I refer below, are Government publications or books which are partially or totally concerned with the National Health Service. Much, however, comes from sources which are not easily available to the student. Journals produced by the many interested groups—to take just two or three examples one may note the *British Medical Journal*, the *County Councils Association Gazette* and *The Hospital* —were relied on heavily in the preparation of this study. Each was, to a greater or lesser extent, the official mouthpiece of an interested group, or at least carried full accounts of the group's views, pronouncements and actions. Allied to this source, I was fortunate in that many of the groups were kind enough to let me see documents which were circulated at various stages among their members. I was further able to discuss many of the points with prominent members of the various groups—one of whom, I discovered, belonged to the group practice with which I was registered. None of these sources is documented in this study, partly because of the complicated referencing this would require and partly because it is hoped that the reader will not concern himself with minute detail but rather see the fuller implications of the history discussed.

The aim of this Note is to draw together the bibliography of a more accessible kind and to direct the interested reader along further lines of exploration for himself. In doing this, it is possible to subdivide the list into three sections :

(A) The Period before 1939

(i) General

The National Health Service developed out of a context of economic and social history, some parts of which are relevant to the subject of this book. It would be wrong to recommend any of the many such books. Instead all I can do is to commend to the reader a good social and economic history of the late nineteenth and early twentieth centuries. This is, I would suggest, a necessary starting point to any further reading on the National Health Service.

(ii) On Health Services

There are few books on the history of health services as a whole : instead books deal with specific events or separate services. Of these the following can be mentioned :

ABEL-SMITH B. *The Hospitals 1800-1948*. Heinemann, London 1964.

A full account of the development of hospitals in this country —a necessary background to any assessment of hospital services today.

WILSON, N. *Municipal Health Services*. Allen and Unwin, London 1947.

An account of pre-1939 local authority health services.

JONES, K. *Lunacy, Law and Conscience—1744-1845*. Routledge and Kegan Paul, London 1955.

Mental Health and Social Policy 1845-1959. Routledge and Kegan Paul, London 1960.

These two accounts of the development of the mental health services are necessary reading for an assessment of this part of the Service.

BRAITHWAITE, W. J. *Lloyd George's Ambulance Wagon*. Methuen, London 1957.

An account by one who played a large part in it, of the negotiations, similar to those discussed in this book, on the National Health Insurance Act, 1911.

HARRIS, R. W. *National Health Insurance 1911 to 1946*. Allen and Unwin, London 1957.

LEVY, H. *National Health Insurance—a critical study*. O.U.P., London 1946.

VERNON, R. V. and MANSBERGH, N. (Eds.) *Advisory Bodies, 1919 to 1939*. Allen and Unwin, London 1940.

This includes references to advisory machinery for pre-1939 services.

NEWSHOLME, SIR A. *Medicine and the State*. Allen and Unwin, London 1932.
P.E.P. *British Health Services*. London 1937.

(B) The Wartime Period

There were many publications during the War, even excluding the group referred to in the first paragraph of this Note, on the National Health Service. The Labour Party, for example, produced the pamphlet *A National Service for Health* in 1943 and the other parties included references to the Service in their literature. Here, however, I want to draw attention to Official publications of this period.

All the following are published by Her Majesty's Stationery Office, London.

Report on Social Insurance and Allied Services Cmd. 6404. 1942.

The Beveridge Report which was to be the blueprint for much of post-war reform and called for, *inter alia*, a comprehensive National Health Service.

Hospital Surveys Nos. 32-264-1 to 10. 1945-6.

These were the products of surveys of hospital facilities and were initiated by the Government in 1941. They make very gloomy reading and perhaps a useful comparative starting point for assessing the achievements of the National Health Service hospitals.

A National Health Service Cmd. 6502. 1944

This is the White Paper discussed in the earlier chapters of this book: it was the first Government plan to be published.

There were three 'Spens' Committees on the remuneration of various professional groups—in each case they were used, to a certain extent, as temporizing devices to circumvent argument. They were:

Report of Inter-Departmental Committee on the Remuneration of General Practitioners Cmd. 6800. 1946.
Report of Inter-Departmental Committee on the Remuneration of Dentists Cmd. 7402. 1948.
Report of Inter-Departmental Committee on the Remuneration of Consultants Cmd. 7420. 1948.

Dentistry posed special problems which were discussed by the 'Teviot' Committee in two reports. They were:

Interim Report of the Inter-Departmental Committee on Dentistry Cmd. 6565. 1944.

Final Report of the Inter-Departmental Committee on Dentistry
Cmd. 6727. 1946.

Finally in this section, one of the Official War Histories must
be highly recommended. It is:

TITMUSS, R. M. *Problems of Social Policy*. H.M.S.O. and Longman
Green and Co., London 1950.

(C) The Period since the 1946 Act
A large number of books have appeared since the Act on the
Service although not many of them can really be recommended.
The explanatory textbook is hard to find and the student would
perhaps do best to refer to textbooks on the Social Services in
general: e.g. D. C. Marsh (Ed.), *Introduction to the Study of Social
Administration*, Routledge and Kegan Paul, London 1965.

The best general surveys to date have both been by American
authors:

LINDSEY, A. *Socialized Medicine in England and Wales*. O.U.P.,
London 1962.
ECKSTEIN, H. *The English Health Service*. O.U.P., London 1959.
The first of these is the better source book, the latter is the
more incisive in its critical assessments. One may also note the
fine study by the second author of the British Medical Association as a pressure group since the Act.
ECKSTEIN, H. *Pressure Group Politics*. Allen and Unwin, London
1960.

This is a case study of the British Medical Association as a
pressure group.

Other books that are worth consulting include:

TITMUSS, R. M. *Essays on the Welfare State*. Allen and Unwin,
London 1958.
TITMUSS, R. M. & ABEL-SMITH, B. *The Cost of the National Health
Service*. O.U.P., 1956.
ROSS, J. S. *The National Health Service in Great Britain*. 1952
O.U.P. 1956.

Among the many publications by Her Majesty's Stationery
Office, in addition to the annual reports of the Minister of Health
and the Central Health Services Council which provide information on the National Health Service, special attention ought to be
directed to:

BIBLIOGRAPHICAL NOTES

The National Health Service (Amendment) Act, 1949.
Enquiry into the Cost of the National Health Service—the Report of the Guillebaud Committee Cmd. 9663. 1956.
Report of the Royal Commission on Doctors and Dentists Remuneration Cmmd. 939. 1960.
Professions (Supplementary to Medicine) Act, 1961.
Social Assay. The Medical Services Review Committee (The 'Porritt' Committee). 1962.

The reader who is interested in making a more detailed analysis of the working of the Service will find helpful articles in such journals as *Medical Care, Sociological Review*, etc. He might look too at the many publications of the Nuffield Provincial Hospitals Trust.

A final note of warning: the National Health Service is now a vast, complicated and expensive service. Comments on it and assessments of it are not easy to make; the reader should therefore beware of the many facile assessments that appear from time to time.